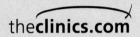

RADIOLOGIC CLINICS

OF NORTH AMERICA

MR Imaging of the Knee

Guest Editor
JEFFREY J. PETERSON, MD

November 2007 • Volume 45 • Number 6

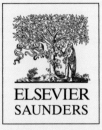

ELSEVIER
SAUNDERS

An imprint of Elsevier, Inc
PHILADELPHIA LONDON TORONTO MONTREAL SYDNEY TOKYO

W.B. SAUNDERS COMPANY
A Division of Elsevier Inc.

1600 John F. Kennedy Boulevard • Suite 1800 • Philadelphia, Pennsylvania 19103-2899

http://www.theclinics.com

RADIOLOGIC CLINICS OF NORTH AMERICA Volume 45, Number 6
November 2007 ISSN 0033-8389; ISBN-13: 978-1-4160-6014-7; ISBN-10: 1-4160-6014-6

Editor: Barton Dudlick

Reprints: For copies of 100 or more, of articles in this publication, please contact the Commercial Reprints Department, Elsevier Inc., 360 Park Avenue South, New York, New York 10010-1710. Tel.: (+1) 212-633-3813; Fax: (+1) 212-462-1935; E-mail: reprints@elsevier.com.

The ideas and opinions expressed in *Radiologic Clinics of North America* do not necessarily reflect those of the Publisher does not assume any responsibility for any injury and/or damage to persons or property arising out of or related to any use of the material contained in this periodical. The reader is advised to check the appropriate medical literature and the product information currently provided by the manufacturer of each drug to be administered to verify the dosage, the method and duration of administration, or contraindications, It is the responsibility of the treating physician or other health care professional, relying on independent experience and knowledge of the patient, to determine drug dosages and the best treatment for the patient. Mention of any product in this issue should not be construed as endorsement by the contributiors, editors, or the Publisher of the productor manufacturers' claims.

Radiologic Clinics of North America (ISSN 0033-8389) is published bimonthly in January, March, May, July, September, and November by Elsevier Inc., 360 Park Avenue South, New York, NY 10010-1710. Business and editorial offices: 1600 John F. Kenedy Boulevard, Suite 1800, Philadelphia, Pennsylvania 19103-2899. Customer Service Office: 6277 Sea Harbor Drive, Orlando, FL 32887-4800. Periodicals postage paid at New York, NY, and additional mailing offices. Subscription prices are USD 290 per year for US individuals, USD 431 per year for US institutions, USD 142 per year for US students and residents, USD 339 per year for Canadian individuals, USD 530 per year of Canadian institutions, USD 394 per year for international individuals, USD 530 per year for international institutions, and USD 192 per year for Canadian and foreign students/residents. To receive student and resident rate, orders must be accompanied by name of affiliated institution, date of term, and the signature of program/residency coordinatior on institution letterhead. Orders will be billed at individual rate until proof of status is received. Foreign air speed delivery is included in all Clinics subscriptionprices. All prices are subject to change without notice. **POSTMASTER:** Send address changes to *Radiologic Clinics of North America*, Elsevier Periodicals Customer Service, 6277 Sea Harbor Drive, Orlando, FL 32887-4800. **Customer Service: 1-800-654-2452 (US). From outside of the US, call (+1) 407-345-4000.**

Radiologic Clinics of North America also published in Greek Paschalidis Medical Publications, Athens, Greece.

Radiologic Clinics of North America is covered in *Index Medicus, EMBASE/Excerpta Medica, Current Contents/Life Sciences, Current Contents/Clinical Medicine, RSNA Index to Imaging Literature, BIOSIS, Science Citation Index,* and *ISI/BIOMED.*

Printed in the United States of America.

MR IMAGING OF THE KNEE

GUEST EDITOR

JEFFREY J. PETERSON, MD
Assistant Professor of Radiology, Department
of Radiology, Mayo Clinic Jacksonville,
Jacksonville, Florida

CONTRIBUTORS

MARK ADKINS, MD
Assistant Professor of Radiology; and Assistant
Professor of Orthopedics, Department of
Radiology, Mayo Clinic and Foundation,
Rochester, Minnesota

LAURA W. BANCROFT, MD
Associate Professor of Radiology, Department of
Radiology, Mayo Clinic, Jacksonville, Florida

FRANCESCA D. BEAMAN, MD
Co-Director of Musculoskeletal Imaging, Center
Radiology, PC, Washington Hospital Center,
Washington, DC

DOUGLAS P. BEALL, MD
Chief of Radiology Services, Clinical Radiology
of Oklahoma; Associate Professor of Orthopedic
Surgery, University of Oklahoma,
Oklahoma City, Oklahoma

THOMAS H. BERQUIST, MD, FACR
Professor, Department of Diagnostic Radiology,
Mayo Clinic College of Medicine, Rochester,
Minnesota; Consultant, Department of Diagnostic
Radiology, Mayo Clinic Jacksonville,
Jacksonville, Florida

JOHN A. CARRINO, MD, MPH
Visiting Associate Professor of Radiology; and
Section Chief, Musculoskeletal Radiology, Russell
H. Morgan Department of Radiology and
Radiological Science, Johns Hopkins University
School of Medicine, Baltimore, Maryland

MICHAEL G. FOX, MD
Assistant Professor, Division of Musculoskeletal
Radiology, Department of Radiology,
University of Virginia, Charlottesville, Virginia

MATTHEW A. FRICK, MD
Instructor, Division of Musculoskeletal
Radiology, Department of Radiology,
Mayo Clinic and Foundation,
Rochester, Minnesota

J. DAVID GOOGE, MD
Department of Orthopedics, University of
Oklahoma Health Science Center,
Oklahoma City, Oklahoma

BARRY J. GREER, MD
Department of Radiology, Wilford Hall Medical
Center, Lackland Air Force Base, Texas

MARK J. KRANSDORF, MD
Professor of Radiology, Mayo Clinic College of
Medicine, Rochester, Minnesota; Consultant,
Mayo Clinic, Jacksonville, Florida

JUSTIN Q. LY, MD
Department of Radiology, Wilford hall Medical
Center, Lackland Air Force Base, Texas

THOMAS MAGEE, MD
Neuroskeletal Imaging, Melbourne, Florida

HAL D. MARTIN, DO
Oklahoma Sports Science & Orthopaedics,
Oklahoma City, Oklahoma

WILLIAM B. MORRISON, MD
Associate Professor of Radiology,
Thomas Jefferson University Hospital,
Philadelphia, Pennsylvania

JASON T. MOSS
Texas Tech University College of Medicine,
Lubbock, Texas

JEFFREY J. PETERSON, MD
Assistant Professor of Radiology, Department
of Radiology, Mayo Clinic Jacksonville,
Jacksonville, Florida

CATHERINE C. ROBERTS, MD
Assistant Professor of Radiology,
Department of Radiology, Mayo Clinic College
of Medicine, Scottsdale, Arizona

MARK J. SPANGEHL, MD
Assistant Professor of Orthopedics, Department of
Orthopedic Surgery, Mayo Clinic College of
Medicine, Scottsdale, Arizona

ANNETTE M. STAPP, RN, BSN
Clinical Radiology of Oklahoma,
Edmond, Oklahoma

JEFFREY D. TOWERS, MD
Chief, Division of Musculoskeletal Imaging,
Department of Radiology, University of Pittsburgh
Medical Center, Pittsburgh, Pennsylvania

DORIS E. WENGER, MD
Assistant Professor of Radiology; and Chair,
Division of Musculoskeletal Imaging, Department
of Radiology, Mayo Clinic and Foundation,
Rochester, Minnesota

MR IMAGING OF THE KNEE

Volume 45 · Number 6 · November 2007

Contents

Laura W. Bancroft

Infectious processes about the knee can result from the hematogenous spread of infection, spread from a contiguous source, direct implantation of pathogens, and prior surgery. Soft tissues, joints, and bones can be infected by bacteria, fungi, parasites, or viruses. MR imaging is useful in identifying cellulitis, abscess, septic arthritis, and osteomyelitis. The inherent tissue contrast provided by MR imaging allows for the delineation of soft-tissue infection and osteomyelitis. Therefore, MR imaging is a useful tool in evaluating the extent of infection, and in facilitating adequate debridement and drainage. MR imaging is particularly useful in the setting of chronic posttraumatic osteomyelitis and in prior surgical procedures, such as arthroscopy, anterior cruciate ligament reconstruction, and amputation.

Mark J. Kransdorf, Jeffrey J. Peterson, and Laura W. Bancroft

The knee joint remains the articulation most frequently assessed by MR imaging, and osseous tumor and tumor-like lesions are not uncommon incidental imaging findings. This article reviews the most commonly encountered incidental lesions, emphasizing the characteristic MR imaging features. It is intended not as a complete review of the imaging findings associated with these lesions but as a summary, highlighting the MR imaging features that are most useful in suggesting a specific diagnosis. The authors organize incidental lesions into the following broad categories: cartilaginous, fibro-osseous, and degenerative. They do not address those lesions that are typically symptomatic and, as a result, likely to be directly related to the patients' clinical presentation and subsequent imaging.

function. MR imaging is accurate and sensitive, making it the imaging technique of choice for evaluating these ligaments. Acute and chronic injuries involving the cruciate ligaments have typical appearances and associated findings. MR imaging interpretation must take into account atypical injuries and imaging pitfalls. Knowledge of normal ligament reconstruction techniques allows differentiation of the normal postoperative appearance from reconstruction failure and complications. Ligament reconstruction techniques, complications, and appearances are reviewed in this article.

Synovial disorders often affect the knee joint and are a common cause of morbidity. Before MR imaging, radiologists were limited in their ability to provide information about the presence or absence of synovial disease. With the advent of MR imaging, useful information can now be provided to referring clinicians, often at a time when the initiation of therapy may mitigate significantly the long-term sequelae of synovial disorders. MR imaging, owing to its superior soft-tissue contrast, is the imaging modality of choice for demonstrating and quantifying pathologic changes of the synovium. MR imaging provides invaluable information to the clinician regarding the need to either initiate or modify therapy in those patients suffering from diseases of, or affecting, the synovium.

MR imaging is the preferred imaging modality for evaluating the meniscus. Overall, when strict criteria are followed, it is accurate in diagnosing meniscal tears in patients who have not had prior meniscal surgery. However, an accurate interpretation requires a through knowledge of the normal meniscal anatomy, common meniscal variants, and common diagnostic pitfalls. In this article, the author emphasizes the importance of describing meniscal tears properly and discusses treatment options. Diagnosing a recurrent tear is more complicated in patients who have had prior partial meniscal resection or repair, and the use of MR arthrography in this group of patients is discussed. Recent developments in areas such as 3 T and parallel imaging offer promise for accurate meniscal evaluation with even shorter scan times.

Three-tesla MR imaging of the knee allows for fast, accurate high-resolution imaging. Three-tesla MR imaging is highly accurate in detection of meniscal tears. This detection aids referring physicians, because if a meniscal tear is not seen on three-tesla MR imaging, it is highly unlikely to be present. High field imaging allows for three-dimensional imaging of the knee. Referring doctors have found this "virtual arthroscopy" to be useful in presurgical planning.

GOAL STATEMENT

The goal of the *Radiologic Clinics of North America* is to keep practicing radiologists and radiology residents up to date with current clinical practice in radiology by providing timely articles reviewing the state of the art in patient care.

ACCREDITATION

The *Radiologic Clinics of North America* is planned and implemented in accordance with the Essential Areas and Policies of the Accreditation Council for Continuing Medical Education (ACCME) through the joint sponsorship of the University of Virginia School of Medicine and Elsevier. The University of Virginia School of Medicine is accredited by the ACCME to provide continuing medical education for physicians.

The University of Virginia School of Medicine designates this educational activity for a maximum of 15 *AMA PRA Category 1 Credits*™. Physicians should only claim credit commensurate with the extent of their participation in the activity.

The American Medical Association has determined that physicians not licensed in the US who participate in this CME activity are eligible for 15 *AMA PRA Category 1 Credits*™.

Credit can be earned by reading the text material, taking the CME examination online at http://www.theclinics.com/home/cme, and completing the evaluation. After taking the test, you will be required to review any and all incorrect answers. Following completion of the test and evaluation, your credit will be awarded and you may print your certificate.

FACULTY DISCLOSURE/CONFLICT OF INTEREST

The University of Virginia School of Medicine, as an ACCME accredited provider, endorses and strives to comply with the Accreditation Council for Continuing Medical Education (ACCME) Standards of Commercial Support, Commonwealth of Virginia statutes, University of Virginia policies and procedures, and associated federal and private regulations and guidelines on the need for disclosure and monitoring of proprietary and financial interests that may affect the scientific integrity and balance of content delivered in continuing medical education activities under our auspices.

The University of Virginia School of Medicine requires that all CME activities accredited through this institution be developed independently and be scientifically rigorous, balanced and objective in the presentation/discussion of its content, theories and practices.

All authors/editors participating in an accredited CME activity are expected to disclose to the readers relevant financial relationships with commercial entities occurring within the past 12 months (such as grants or research support, employee, consultant, stock holder, member of speakers bureau, etc.). The University of Virginia School of Medicine will employ appropriate mechanisms to resolve potential conflicts of interest to maintain the standards of fair and balanced education to the reader. Questions about specific strategies can be directed to the Office of Continuing Medical Education, University of Virginia School of Medicine, Charlottesville, Virginia.

The authors/editors listed below have identified no financial or professional relationships for themselves or their spouse/partner:
Mark Adkins, MD; Francesca D. Beaman, MD; Thomas H. Berquist, MD, FACR; John A. Carrino, MD, MPH; Barton Dudlick (Acquisitions Editor); Michael G. Fox, MD; Matthew A. Frick, MD: J. David Googe, MD; Barry J. Greer, MD; Justin Q. Ly, MD; Thomas Magee, MD; Hal D. Martin, DO; William B. Morrison, MD; Jason T. Moss; Jeffrey J. Peterson, MD (Guest Editor); Catherine C. Roberts, MD; Annette M. Stapp, RN, BSN; Jeffrey D. Towers, MD; and, Doris E. Wenger, MD.

The authors/editors listed below have identified the following financial or professional relationships for themselves or their spouse/partner:
Laura W. Bancroft, MD is a speaker for Ryals and Associates.
Douglas P. Beall, MD is an independent contractor, a consultant, on the Speaker's Bureau, and on the Advisory Committee for Medtronic, is an independent contractor, a consultant, and on the Speaker's Bureau for Kyphon; is an independent contractor, a consultant, on the Speaker's Bureau, on the Advisory Committe, and owns stock in Spineology; and, is a consultant and on the Speaker's Bureau for Lilly.
Mark J. Kransdorf, MD is a speaker for Ryals and Associates; and is an author for Lippincott, Williams & Wilkins, and Elsevier.
Mark J. Spengehl, MD is on the Advisory Committee for Depuy Orthopaedics.

Disclosure of Discussion of Non-FDA Approved Uses for Pharmaceutical and/or Medical Devices:
The University of Virginia School of Medicine, as an ACCME provider, requires that all authors identify and disclose any "off label" uses for pharmaceutical and medical device products. The University of Virginia School of Medicine recommends that each physician fully review all the available data on new products or procedures prior to clinical use.

TO ENROLL

To enroll in the *Radiologic Clinics of North America* Continuing Medical Education program, call customer service at 1-800-654-2452 or sign up online at http://www.theclinics.com/home/cme. The CME program is available to subscribers for an additional annual fee USD 205.

RADIOLOGIC CLINICS OF NORTH AMERICA

Radiol Clin N Am 45 (2007) xi

Preface

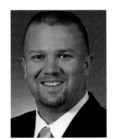

Jeffrey J. Peterson, MD
Guest Editor

Jeffrey J. Peterson, MD
Assistant Professor of Radiology
Department of Radiology
Mayo Clinic Jacksonville
4500 San Pablo Road
Jacksonville, FL 32224, USA

E-mail address:
peterson.jeffrey@mayo.edu

I hope the reader will enjoy this issue of *Radiologic Clinics of North America*, which focuses on the current applications of MR imaging of the knee joint. MR imaging has had a remarkable impact on musculoskeletal imaging, and imaging of the knee for evaluation of internal derangement continues to be one of the most frequently performed examinations. This issue offers a thorough and insightful review of the anatomy and pathophysiology of the knee, and highlights many of the recent advances in knowledge and technology in regards to knee joint MR imaging. This issue also provides an up-to-date review of the various imaging sequences and techniques that can be useful for the evaluation of specific structures of the knee joint, and presents an enlightening update on methods to optimize image quality and MR performance. It seems every year that we more fully understand the anatomy and the mechanics of knee joint injuries, and with continued advances in technology and sequence design, MR imaging reveals both the anatomy and the pathology of the knee joint with more precision and detail than previously possible.

I would like to express my sincere gratitude to the contributing authors for their exceptional work. Many long hours went into the preparation of each of these articles, and I would like to thank my colleagues for readily sharing their expertise. I would also like to thank Barton Dudlick and the remainder of the staff at Elsevier for their assistance on this issue. We hope you find the issue informative and educational, and a helpful resource for interpreting MR examinations of the knee.

This article was originally published in *Magnetic Resonance Imaging Clinics of North America* 15:1, February 2007.

doi:10.1016/j.rcl.2007.08.011
radiologic.theclinics.com

RADIOLOGIC
CLINICS
OF NORTH AMERICA

Radiol Clin N Am 45 (2007) 931–941

MR Imaging of Infectious Processes of the Knee

Laura W. Bancroft, MD

Infectious processes about the knee can result from the hematogenous spread of infection from remote sources, spread from a contiguous source of infection, direct implantation of pathogens, and prior surgery [1]. Soft tissues, joints, and bones are infected most commonly by bacteria, although a few cases are caused by fungi, parasites, or viruses. MR imaging is useful in identifying cellulitis, abscess, septic arthritis, and osteomyelitis. MR imaging is particularly useful in the setting of chronic posttraumatic osteomyelitis and in prior surgical procedures, such as arthroscopy, anterior cruciate ligament (ACL) reconstruction, and amputation.

Soft-tissue infection

Soft-tissue infection about the knee can occur either primarily (with or without secondary extension to the bone or joint) (Fig. 1) or secondarily, from extension of an intraosseous or intra-articular infection. Cellulitis is a term denoting infection localized to the subcutaneous tissues. MR imaging will demonstrate a reticulated pattern of abnormal signal intensity in the subcutaneous tissue on both T1-weighted and fluid-sensitive sequences (see

Fig. 1). If intravenous contrast is administered, the subcutaneous tissues will have a reticulated pattern of enhancement. In comparison, noninfective edema may have similar signal characteristics but will fail to enhance.

Fasciitis occurs when infection involves the deep or superficial fascia. Soft-tissue gas is a useful radiographic and CT imaging feature that is suggestive of necrotizing fasciitis. However, MR imaging is less sensitive than CT for the detection of soft-tissue gas. Hyperintense T2-weighted signal within deep fascial planes and muscle, with or without enhancement, can be seen in necrotizing soft-tissue infection and other conditions [2].

Pyomyositis tends to involve the large muscles of the lower extremity, and is caused by *Staphylococcus aureus* in about 90% of cases [3]. Patient factors that increase the risk of pyomyositis include diabetes mellitus, HIV, chronic steroid use, connective tissue disorders, malignancy, and multiple hematologic disorders [3]. Pyomyositis may also occur as a result of iatrogenic inoculation from various surgical procedures or contiguous spread of infection from adjacent soft tissues, bones, or joints. MR imaging demonstrates increased signal intensity in the

This article was originally published in *Magnetic Resonance Imaging Clinics of North America* 15:1, February 2007.

Department of Radiology, Mayo Clinic, 4500 San Pablo Road, Jacksonville, FL 32224-3899, USA
E-mail address: bancroft.laura@mayo.edu

doi:10.1016/j.rcl.2007.08.002

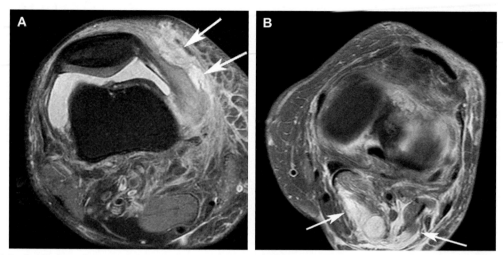

Fig. 1. Periarticular soft-tissue infection. (*A*) Axial proton density fat-suppressed image in a 38-year-old diabetic man demonstrates fluid (*arrows*) superficial to the vastus medialis, diffuse cellulitis, and a small joint effusion. Culture of the drained abscess revealed *Staphylococcus aureus*. (*B*) Axial proton density fat-suppressed image in a 71-year-old woman demonstrates complex fluid in the popliteal fossa (*arrows*) that insinuates throughout the posterior compartment musculature around the neurovascular bundle. Aspiration revealed *Streptococcus viridans* and patient subsequently developed septic arthritis.

muscle on fluid-sensitive sequences. If an intramuscular abscess is present, it is hyperintense on fluid-sensitive sequences, and the rim can be increased in signal on T1-weighted images and decreased on T2-weighted images, and can enhance with intravenous gadolinium (Fig. 2) [3]. Pyomyositis also may be associated with cellulitis, which can help differentiate pyomyositis from other benign or malignant soft-tissue masses [3]. Knee joint effusions distal to, and separate from, the site of muscle infection may be sympathetic and not septic [3].

Septic arthritis

Septic arthritis indicates an infectious process localized to the joint. Although no single MR imaging feature can differentiate septic from nonseptic arthritis, the presence of several abnormal findings can increase the probability of infection. Concomitant bone erosions and marrow edema are highly suggestive of septic arthritis, and the added presence of synovial thickening, synovial edema, soft-tissue edema, or bone marrow enhancement is even more suggestive of infection (Fig. 3) [4]. Joint effusions are nonspecific findings, and can be present in both septic and nonseptic joints. Furthermore, up to one third of patients who have septic arthritis can lack a joint effusion [5]. Abnormal marrow signal is worrisome for concomitant osteomyelitis, especially if diffuse and identified on T1-weighted images [5].

Osteomyelitis

Osteomyelitis is an infection of the bone and marrow that is usually the result of a bacterial infection, although it may be caused by fungi, parasites, and viruses [1]. Resnick [1] uses the term infective (suppurative) osteitis to indicate isolated contamination of cortical bone, which can occur separately from, or, more commonly, in conjunction with, osteomyelitis. Infective (suppurative) periostitis indicates involvement of the periosteum only [1].

Osteomyelitis is caused by the hematogenous spread of infection or is spread from a contiguous source, including direct implantation (eg, puncture wound, surgery) or extension from an adjacent infection (eg, skin, soft tissue, joint) [6]. Hematogenous osteomyelitis typically affects the metaphysis of tubular bones [1,7]. Direct penetration or implantation (contiguous-focus) is now the most common cause of osteomyelitis in the United States [7]. Osteomyelitis is classified as acute, subacute, or chronic, depending on the rate of onset and the intensity of the associated symptoms [1,6].

Acute osteomyelitis

Acute osteomyelitis is an acute, suppurative infection [1,6]. Typically, acute hematogenous osteomyelitis is considered a disease of children, usually between 3 and 15 years old [1,7]. Hematogenous osteomyelitis most commonly involves the

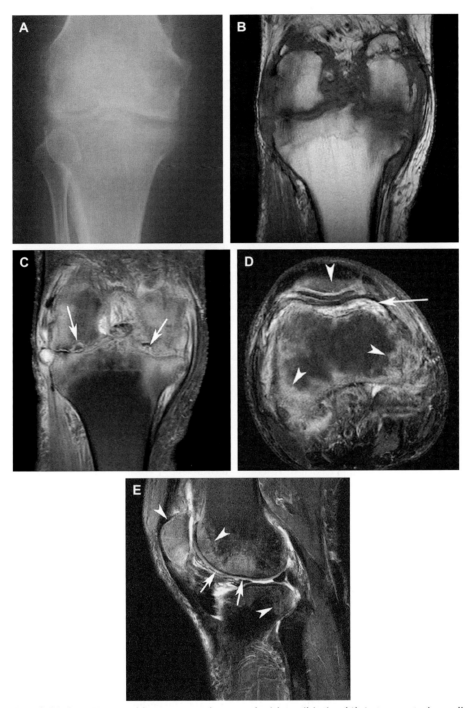

Fig. 2. Septic arthritis in a 58-year-old man currently treated with antibiotics. (*A*) Anteroposterior radiograph of the knee demonstrates generalized joint space narrowing, subchondral sclerosis, and erosions. (*B*) Coronal T1-weighted image demonstrates extensive changes of septic arthritis, with diffuse chondrolysis, subchondral erosions, hypointense marrow signal intensity in the subarticular tibia and femur, and abnormal periarticular soft tissue. (*C*) Coronal FSE T2-weighted fat-suppressed image demonstrates fluid within the osteochondral defects (*arrows*) and multiple subcortical erosions. (*D*) Axial FSE proton density fat-suppressed image delineates the extent of marrow edema-like signal throughout the patella and femur (*arrowheads*), and the thickened synovium (*arrow*). (*E*) Sagittal FSE T2-weighted fat-suppressed image delineates the chondrolysis (*arrows*) and periarticular marrow edema-like signal (*arrowheads*).

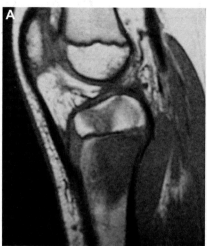 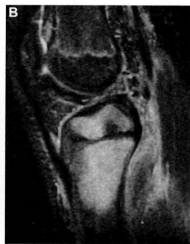

Fig. 3. Osteomyelitis in the proximal tibial metaphysis with spread across the physis in an 8-year-old girl. (*A*) T1-weighted sagittal image demonstrates abnormal hypointense signal intensity, predominantly in the proximal tibial metaphysis, with transphyseal extension into the epiphysis. (*B*) Fast short tau inversion recovery (STIR) sagittal image demonstrates abnormal hyperintense signal intensity in a slightly larger distribution than the T1-weighted images, consistent with marrow edema-like signal from osteomyelitis.

metaphyses of tubular bones in children, but it can involve flat or irregularly shaped bones in up to 25% of cases [1]. An adjacent joint effusion is present in about 60% of cases [6]. Extensive involucrum formation is also characteristic of osteomyelitis in infants because the periosteum can be separated easily from the adjacent bone [1].

MR imaging can identify the presence of osteomyelitis and determine the degree of involvement. The affected marrow shows poorly marginated areas of abnormal signal intensity, with decreased signal intensity on T1-weighted images and corresponding increased signal intensity on fluid-sensitive images (see Fig. 3) [8]. Cortical signal is preserved in early cases [8]; however, with time, abnormal signal will extend into the cortex, the periosteum, and soft tissue. Erdman and colleagues [8] found MR imaging to be 100% sensitive for bacterial osteomyelitis, with a specificity of 75% to 82%; the specificity was decreased because of other causes of abnormal signal intensity, such as septic joint, fracture, or infarction. Abnormal signal on short tau inversion recovery (STIR) sequences typically overestimates the true extent of the infected marrow [9]. Before abscess formation, involved tissue shows enhancement following contrast administration, reflecting the inflammatory nature of the underlying process, with almost all-enhancing marrow reflecting areas of active infection [9]. An abscess may also show more well-defined margins on T2-weighted images, and a rind of decreased signal [10]. Contrast-enhanced imaging is especially helpful in differentiating an abscess from diffuse

inflammation, both of which may show increased signal intensity on fluid-sensitive sequences.

Subacute osteomyelitis

Brodie's abscess, also referred to as "cystic" osteomyelitis, is a specific form of osteomyelitis that can occur in either subacute or chronic infection (Fig. 4) [7,11]. Typically, it is seen in young men, with 75% of patients under 25 years old [7]. The cause of this form of osteomyelitis is unknown, but it may arise spontaneously in association with a focal inflammatory episode, or after hematogenous infection [7]. Radiographically, Brodie's abscess is a geographic lesion with a well-defined sclerotic margin, located in the metaphysis. A radiolucent channel, representing a sinus tract, may be seen, which can communicate with the physis [1,7].

MR imaging demonstrates a Brodie's abscess as a well-defined lesion that is hypointense to marrow on T1-weighted images and hyperintense on fluid-sensitive sequences. The margin of the abscess may be either hypointense or hyperintense. The penumbra sign is a characteristic MR imaging feature of subacute osteomyelitis that represents a thin layer of granulation tissue that lines the abscess cavity [12,13]. The penumbra sign is identified on unenhanced T1-weighted images as a discrete peripheral zone of slightly increased signal intensity, relative to the central abscess cavity and the surrounding hypointense reactive new bone and edema [12], and is often present about the knee in either the distal femur or proximal tibia.

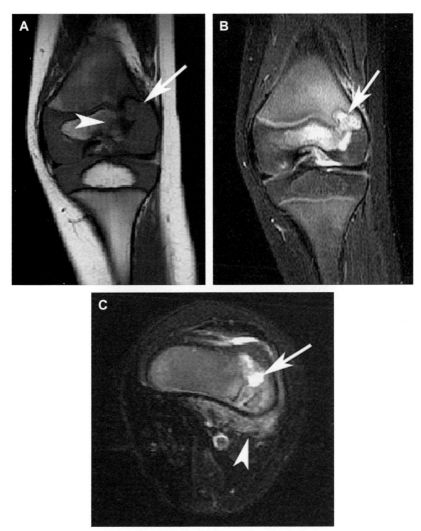

Fig. 4. Subacute osteomyelitis with a Brodie's abscess. Coronal T1-weighted (*A*) and STIR (*B*) images demonstrate extension of a Brodie's abscess (*arrow*) across the physis, into the metaphysis. Note the prolonged T1 and T2 relaxation time in the mid- and lateral epiphyseal marrow (*arrowhead*) and the distal femoral metaphysis, consistent with edema-like signal from osteomyelitis. (*C*) Axial STIR image through the distal femoral metaphysis demonstrates the hyperintense Brodie's abscess (*arrow*), diffusely abnormal metaphyseal marrow signal, and marked periosteal thickening (*arrowhead*).

Chronic osteomyelitis

Chronic osteomyelitis occurs when there is a residual nidus of infection and a refractory clinical course [1,6]. Chronic osteomyelitis is the result of continuous infection or reactivation, usually by a low-virulence organism [7]. After a period of inactivity, lesions may become active. Chronic osteomyelitis is frequently the result of long-standing indolent infection, often as a result of inappropriate or inadequate treatment, and has a predilection for the metaphyses of long bones [7].

MR imaging of chronic osteomyelitis often reveals a thickened cortex with a sharp interface between involved and uninvolved marrow, and well-defined, associated soft-tissue abnormality [8,14]. A rim of decreased signal, presumably representing fibrous tissue, may also surround areas of chronic active infection (Fig. 5) [8]. Usually, osseous remodeling is identified, and disruption of cortical bone and sinus tracts may be seen also [8]. Sinus tracts typically extend to cutaneous ulcers, and often are seen overlying weight-bearing prominences [9]. On MR imaging, metaphyseal disease may be obscured by adjacent hematopoietic marrow on T1-weighted images [15]. T2-weighted images and STIR images usually show less signal intensity in normal hematopoietic marrow than in marrow infiltrated by infectious exudate [15]. Although usually present, bone marrow edema may not be

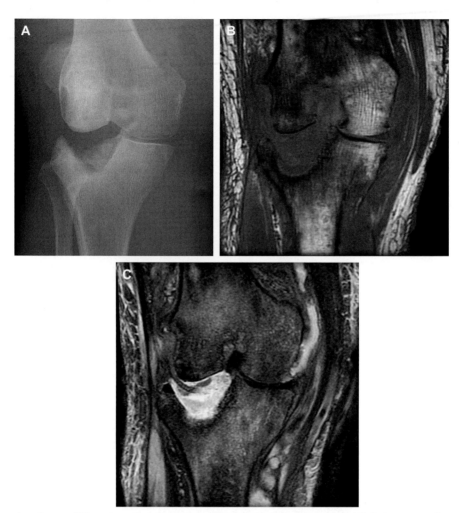

Fig. 5. Chronic osteomyelitis and septic arthritis in a 60-year-old diabetic woman. (*A*) Anteroposterior radiograph demonstrates a large defect within the lateral tibial plateau, with a well-marginated contour and extensive sclerosis. Coronal images through the knee demonstrate extensive changes of chronic osteomyelitis and septic arthritis, with areas of marrow edema that are nearly isointense to muscle on T1-weighted image (*B*) and slightly hyperintense to muscle on FSE T2-weighted fat-suppressed image (*C*). Note that the large lateral tibial defect is filled with joint fluid, and the complex fluid tracking medial and lateral to the knee joint. Surgery showed gross pyarthrosis, which cultured group B *Streptococcus*.

detected if sclerosis is surrounding a bone abscess [16]. Fast inversion-recovery sequences may be more sensitive than fast spin-echo (FSE) sequences for the detection of abnormal marrow [17].

Umans and colleagues [18] reported the usefulness of intravenous gadolinium for the differentiation of osteomyelitis from bone infarction in patients who were at risk for both processes. Patients who have osteomyelitis have more geographic and irregular marrow enhancement on enhanced MR imaging, compared with the thin, linear rim enhancement associated with acute bone infarcts [18]. In addition, osteomyelitis may demonstrate subtle cortical defects with abnormal signal traversing marrow and soft tissue [18].

Chronic post-traumatic osteomyelitis

The evaluation of active osteomyelitis in the setting of chronic posttraumatic osteomyelitis can be difficult; however, acute activity in chronic osteomyelitis can be excluded with high likelihood if the MR imaging findings are negative [19]. Pitfalls occur because reparative fibrovascular scar tissue in the bone marrow and traumatized soft tissue can persist for up to a year after surgical intervention [19,20]. In addition, heterogeneously hypo- and hyperintense osseous signal can be evident on fluid-sensitive sequences after trauma, limiting the detection of superimposed infection. Ledermann and colleagues [20] reported 63% specificity and 100% sensitivity

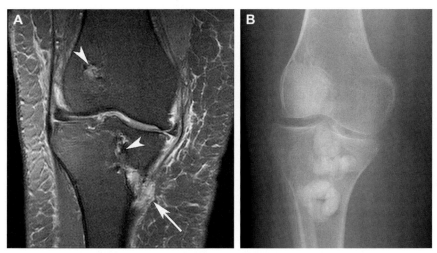

Fig. 6. Infected ACL graft requiring removal in a 43-year-old woman. (*A*) Coronal T1-weighed enhanced fat-suppressed image through the knee demonstrates abnormal enhancement (*arrow*) surrounding the intact ACL graft (*arrowheads*). (*B*) Anteroposterior radiograph of the knee demonstrates antibiotic-laden cement in the ACL tunnel, after infected graft removal.

of enhanced MR imaging for the diagnosis of relapsing, active osteomyelitis in the setting of chronic posttraumatic osteomyelitis. In chronic posttraumatic osteomyelitis, the presence of soft-tissue sinus tracts increases the likelihood of infection [20]. However, cutaneous ulcerations and cortical irregularities are not specific for the presence or absence of infection in the setting of prior trauma [19,20]. Gadolinium may be helpful in differentiating abscess from diffuse inflammatory

change, and fibrovascular scar from infectious foci, in the setting of chronic posttraumatic osteomyelitis [19,20].

Postoperative knee infection

Anterior cruciate ligament reconstruction

Postoperative infection of the knee is uncommon after arthroscopy, ACL reconstruction, or arthroplasty

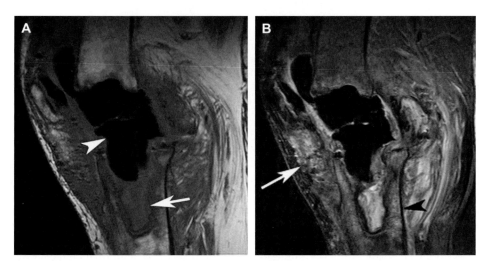

Fig. 7. Cement spacer after removal of chronically infected total knee arthroplasty in a 76-year-old woman. (*A*) Sagittal T1-weighted image demonstrates an intra-articular signal void (*arrowhead*), corresponding to antibiotic-impregnated cement spacer placed after removal of infected total knee arthroplasty. Note the proximal tibial defect (*arrow*) previously occupied by the knee arthroplasty, and the abnormal hypointense signal throughout the adjacent soft tissues. (*B*) Sagittal FSE T2-weighted image redemonstrates the articular spacer, the complex fluid within the tibial defect, and the abnormally increased signal within the proximal tibia marrow (*arrow*), consistent with osteomyelitis. Note the extensively abnormal extraosseous soft tissues (*arrow*), consistent with soft-tissue infection.

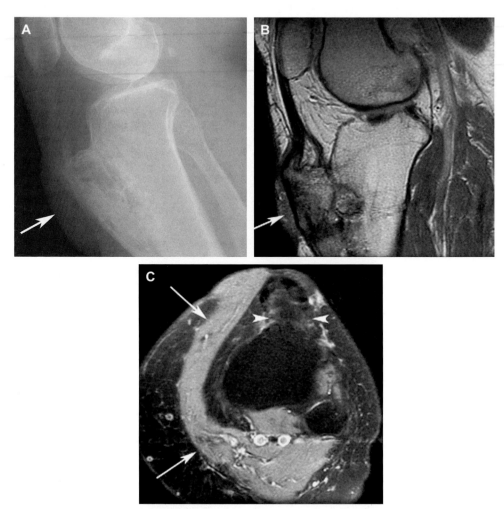

Fig. 8. Myocutaneous flap coverage for tibial osteomyelitis in a 45-year-old woman. (*A*) Lateral radiograph demonstrates pretibial soft tissue corresponding to the myocutaneous flap (*arrow*), which was placed for soft-tissue coverage after osteomyelitis, complicating the anterior tubercle elevation performed for patellofemoral arthritis (Maquet's procedure). Sagittal proton density (*B*) and axial proton density fat-suppressed (*C*) images demonstrate the rotated medial head of the gastrocnemius (*arrows*) into the pretibial soft-tissue defect. Note the healed tibial tubercle elevation (*arrowheads*).

[21]. The incidence of postoperative infection after all arthroscopic procedures is reported to be between 0.1% to 0.4% [22]. The incidence of infection after arthroscopic ACL reconstruction ranges between 0.3% and 1% [22–25]. When autologous patellar or quadriceps tendons are used for graft reconstruction, the grafted portion of the knee and the donor site may become infected. Strict quality measures are maintained at licensed donor banks, which severely limit the incidence of transmittable bacteria and viruses in ACL autografts. However, undetected contamination can occur while harvesting, storing, or manipulating the graft before implantation. Diaz-de-Rada and colleagues [26] reported that 13% of 118 patients who had cadaveric-bone–patellar-bone allografts had positive cultures, but no clinical signs of infection.

Although arthrocentesis is required to diagnose infection, MR imaging may be helpful in the diagnosis or exclusion of infection (Fig. 6). Because the ACL graft is avascular, it normally does not demonstrate enhancement. An infected ACL graft may be focally or diffusely hyperintense, likely because of fibrinous exudate on its surface [23]. However, noninfected periligamentous tissues are normally higher in signal intensity, and can enhance because of their vascularity and developing granulation tissue or immature collagen [27].

Although nonspecific for infection, joint effusion, synovitis, and edema of the adjacent soft tissue and bone marrow can occur in the setting of infection after ACL grafting [23,28]. Osseous erosions, sinus tracts, and soft-tissue abscesses are more specific signs of musculoskeletal infection

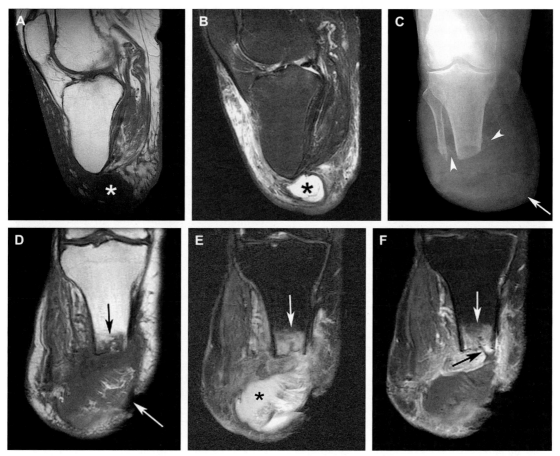

Fig. 9. Recurrent abscess and development of osteomyelitis after below-knee amputation in an 80-year-old woman with peripheral vascular disease. Sagittal T1-weighted (*A*) and FSE T2-weighted fat-suppressed (*B*) images demonstrate a well-defined fluid collection (*) with a thick border distal to the tibial stump, which proved to be an abscess. The underlying bone maintains its hypointense margin and normal marrow signal intensity. Patient underwent debridement of the abscess. (*C*) Anteroposterior radiograph obtained 13 months later depicts new periosteal reaction about the stump (*arrowheads*) and soft-tissue ulceration about the medial, distal soft tissues (*arrow*). (*D*) Coronal T1-weighted image defines the depth of the ulceration (*white arrow*) and new, abnormal, hypointense marrow signal (*black arrow*) within the tibial centimeter of the stump. (*E*) FSE T2-weighted fat-suppressed image demonstrates myonecrosis and progressive abscess (*) within the distal stump. Note the marrow edema-like signal within the stump (*arrow*). (*F*) Enhanced T1-weighted fat-suppressed image demonstrates communication of the abscess with the distal stump (*black arrow*), leading to contiguous spread of infection to the bone (*white arrow*).

on MR imaging. Osteomyelitis should be suspected when MR imaging shows replaced marrow fat-signal on T1-weighted images and more intense marrow enhancement. However, intra-tunnel ganglia, cysts, and surrounding bone marrow edema-like signal may be present in the setting of noninfected ACL reconstructions [27,29].

Periprosthetic infection

Multiple complications can occur after knee arthroplasty, including aseptic loosening, periprosthetic and patellar fracture, extensor mechanism

abnormalities, component failure, peroneal nerve palsy, prolonged serous drainage, and infection [30,31]. With the development of improved orthopedic techniques and antibiotics, the rate of deep infection after primary total knee arthroplasty is currently less than 1%, and wound infection after revision arthroplasty is less than 2% [32,33]. The diagnosis of infection is based most commonly on a combination of clinical findings (pain, redness, swelling, elevated erythrocyte sedimentation rate, C-reactive protein, and leukocytosis), radiographs, aspiration cultures, and scintigraphy. Radiography is not reliable in the diagnosis or exclusion of infection after arthroplasty; however, endosteal scalloping, laminated periosteal reaction, sequestra, and intra-articular gas are fairly specific radiographic signs for infection [34]. Ill-defined periprosthetic resorption, acute periosteal reaction, and multiple foci of subacute periosteal reaction are also highly worrisome for osteomyelitis [35].

MR imaging is used rarely for the evaluation of periprosthetic infection. Distortion and image degradation related to the metallic prostheses can hinder significantly the evaluation of anatomic imaging with MR imaging, depending on the type of metal and MR imaging techniques used [36,37]. Titanium implants usually result in less metallic artifact than stainless steel, allowing more of the adjacent bone and soft tissue to be evaluated [37]. Prostheses that are fairly linear and uniform in their construction result in fewer artifacts than implants that are rounded or irregular [37]. The use of several MR imaging techniques also reduces the amount of field-inhomogeneity artifact generated by metallic implants. These techniques include designating the frequency-encoding direction along the long axis of the prosthesis, increasing the frequency-encoding gradient strength, using FSE sequences, increasing the echo train length and increasing readout bandwidth [37,38]. Furthermore, chemical fat saturation and gradient-echo imaging should be avoided because they result in greater artifact [37,39].

MR imaging can be useful in the evaluation of persistent infection after explantation because focal intraosseous and soft-tissue abscesses can be well visualized. Antibiotic-laden cement usually presents as a signal void with very little artifact on MR imaging (Fig. 7).

Myocutaneous flap

In the event of infection, myocutaneous flaps may be required for adequate soft-tissue coverage after debridement of soft tissue or bone (Fig. 8) [40]. Flaps about the knee may be rotational flaps, commonly obtained from the gastrocnemius muscle, but can also be free flaps from distant sites. These autografts resemble muscle on MR imaging, but may have an edema-like signal within them. Myocutaneous flaps also develop progressive fatty atrophy on sequential MR imaging [40].

Amputation

Patients requiring either above- or below-knee amputations for osteomyelitis may require further intervention because of either residual or recurrent soft-tissue or osseous infection. MR imaging can detect stump abscesses readily (Fig. 9), thereby facilitating either image-guided or surgical drainage. If the infection progresses to involve the osseous stump, MR imaging is useful in delineating the extent of osteomyelitis before surgical debridement.

Summary

MR imaging is useful in identifying cases of cellulitis, fasciitis, abscess, septic arthritis, and osteomyelitis about the knee. The inherent tissue contrast provided by MR imaging allows for the delineation of soft-tissue infection and osteomyelitis. Therefore, MR imaging is a useful tool in evaluating the extent of infection, and in facilitating adequate debridement and drainage. MR imaging can be particularly useful in complicated settings, such as chronic posttraumatic osteomyelitis, and in postsurgical patients after arthroscopy, ACL reconstruction, and amputation.

References

[1] Resnick D. Osteomyelitis, septic arthritis, and soft tissue infection: mechanisms and situations. In: Resnick D, editor. Diagnosis of bone and joint disorders. 4th edition. Philadelphia: WB Saunders; 2002. p. 2377–480.

[2] Loh NN, Ch'en IY, Cheung LP, et al. Deep fascial hyperintensity in soft-tissue abnormalities as revealed by T2-weighted MR imaging. AJR Am J Roentgenol 1997;168:1301–4.

[3] Gordon BA, Martinez S, Collins AJ. Pyomyositis: characteristics at CT and MR imaging. Radiology 1995;197:279–86.

[4] Graif M, Schweitzer ME, Deely D, et al. The septic versus nonseptic inflamed joint: MRI characteristics. Skeletal Radiol 1999;28:616–20.

[5] Karchevsky M, Schweitzer ME, Morrison WB, et al. MRI findings of septic arthritis and associated osteomyelitis in adults. AJR Am J Roentgenol 2004;182:119–22.

[6] Mader JT, Calhoun J. Osteomyelitis. In: Mandell GL, Bennett JE, Dolin R, editors. Principles and practice of infectious disease. 5th edition. Philadelphia: Churchill Livingstone; 2000. p. 1182–200.

[7] David R, Barrow BJ, Madwell JE. Osteomyelitis, acute and chronic. Radiol Clin North Am 1987; 25:1171–202.

[8] Erdman WA, Tamburro F, Jayson HT, et al. Osteomyelitis: characteristics and pitfalls of diagnosis with MR imaging. Radiology 1991;180:533–9.

[9] Deely MD, Schweitzer ME. MR imaging of bone marrow disorders. Radiol Clin North Am 1997; 35:193–212.

[10] Schlesinger AE, Hernandez RJ. Diseases of the musculoskeletal system in children: imaging with CT, sonography, and MR. AJR Am J Roentgenol 1992;158:729–41.

[11] Brodie BC. An account of some cases of chronic abscess of the tibia. Medico-Chirurgical Transactions 1832;17:239–49.

[12] Davies AM, Grimer R. The penumbra sign in subacute osteomyelitis. Eur Radiol 2005;15: 1268–70.

[13] Grey AC, Davies AM, Mangham DC, et al. The "penumbra sign" on T1-weighted MR imaging in subacute osteomyelitis: frequency, cause and significance. Clin Radiol 1998;53:587–92.

[14] Cohen MD, Cory DA, Kleiman M, et al. Magnetic resonance differentiation of acute and chronic osteomyelitis in children. Clin Radiol 1990;41:53–6.

[15] Jaramillo D, Treves ST, Kasser JR, et al. Osteomyelitis and septic arthritis in children: appropriate use of imaging to guide treatment. AJR Am J Roentgenol 1995;165:399–404.

[16] Wingen M, Alzen G, Gunther RW. MR imaging fails to detect bone marrow oedema in osteomyelitis: report of two cases. Pediatr Radiol 1998; 28:189–92.

[17] Hauer MP, Uhl M, Allmann KH, et al. Comparison of turbo inversion recovery magnitude (TIRM) with T2-weighted turbo spin-echo and T1-weighted spin-echo MR imaging in the early diagnosis of acute osteomyelitis in children. Pediatr Radiol 1998;28:846–50.

[18] Umans H, Haramati N, Flusser G. The diagnostic role of gadolinium enhanced MRI in distinguishing between acute medullary bone infarct and osteomyelitis. Magn Reson Imaging 2000;18: 255–62.

[19] Kaim AH, Gross T, von Schulthess GK. Imaging of chronic posttraumatic osteomyelitis. Eur Radiol 2002;12:1193–202.

[20] Ledermann HP, Kaim A, Bongartz G, et al. Pitfalls and limitations of magnetic resonance imaging in chronic posttraumatic osteomyelitis. Eur Radiol 2000;10:1815–23.

[21] Anract P, Missenard G, Jeanrot C, et al. Knee reconstruction with prosthesis and muscle flap after total arthrectomy. Clin Orthop Relat Res 2001;384:208–16.

[22] Burks RT, Friederichs MG, Fink B, et al. Treatment of postoperative anterior cruciate ligament infections with graft removal and early reimplantation. Am J Sports Med 2003;31:414–8.

[23] Papakonstantinou O, Chung CB, Chanchairujira K, et al. Complications of anterior cruciate ligament reconstruction: MR imaging. Eur Radiol 2003;13: 1106–17.

[24] Zalavras CG, Patzakis MJ, Tibone J, et al. Treatment of persistent infection after anterior cruciate ligament surgery. Clin Orthop Relat Res 2005;439:52–5.

[25] Fong SY. Septic arthritis after arthroscopic anterior cruciate ligament reconstruction. Ann Acad Med Singapore 2004;33:228–34.

[26] Diaz-de-Rada P, Barriga A, Barrosa JL, et al. Positive culture in allograft ACL-reconstruction: what to do? Knee Surg Sports Traumatol Arthrosc 2003;11:219–22.

[27] Jansson KA, Karjalainen PT, Harilainen A, et al. MRI of anterior cruciate ligament repair with patellar and hamstring tendon autografts. Skeletal Radiol 2001;30:8–14.

[28] Bach FD, Carlier JB, Elis JB, et al. Anterior cruciate ligament reconstruction with bioabsorbable polyglycolic acid interference screws: MR imaging follow-up. Radiology 2002;225:541–50.

[29] McCauley TR. MR imaging evaluation of the postoperative knee. Radiology 2004;234:53–61.

[30] Taljanovic MS, Jones MD, Hunter TB, et al. Joint arthroplasties and prostheses. Radiographics 2003;23:1295–314.

[31] Ayers DC, Dennis DA, Johanson NA, et al. Common complications of total knee arthroplasty. J Bone Joint Surg Am 1997;79:278–304.

[32] SooHoo NF, Lieberman JR, Ko CY, et al. Factors predicting complication rates following total knee replacement. J Bone Joint Surg Am 2006; 8:480–5.

[33] Mahomed NN, Barrett J, Katz JN, et al. Epidemiology of total knee replacement in the United States Medicare population. J Bone Joint Surg Am 2005;87:1222–8.

[34] Lyons CW, Berquist TH, Lyons JC, et al. Evaluation of radiographic findings in painful hip arthroplasties. Clin Orthop 1985;195:239–51.

[35] Bauer T, Schils J. The pathology of total joint arthoplasty: II. Mechanisms of implant failure. Skeletal Radiol 1999;28:483–97.

[36] Frick MA, Collins MS, Adkins MC. Postoperative imaging of the knee. Radiol Clin North Am 2006;44:367–89.

[37] Sofka CM. Optimizing techniques for musculoskeletal imaging of the postoperative patient. Radiol Clin North Am 2006;44:323–9.

[38] Peterson JJ. Postoperative infection. Radiol Clin North Am 2006;44:439–50.

[39] Math KR, Zaidi SF, Petchprapa C, et al. Imaging of total knee arthroplasty. Semin Musculoskelet Radiol 2006;10:47–62.

[40] Fox MG, Bancroft LW, Peterson JJ, et al. MRI appearance of myocutaneous flaps commonly used in orthopedic reconstructive surgery. AJR Am J Roentgenol 2006;187:800–6.

ELSEVIER
SAUNDERS

RADIOLOGIC
CLINICS
OF NORTH AMERICA

Radiol Clin N Am 45 (2007) 943–954

MR Imaging of the Knee: Incidental Osseous Lesions

Mark J. Kransdorf, MD[a,b,]*, Jeffrey J. Peterson, MD[c],
Laura W. Bancroft, MD[c]

- Radiographs
- Common incidental lesions
  Cartilaginous tumors
  Fibro-osseous lesions

Degenerative lesions
- Summary
- References

The knee remains one of the most commonly imaged articulations. Consequently, tumor or tumor-like lesions are not uncommon incidental findings. Unlike patients who present specifically for the evaluation of a mass, individuals who have incidentally identified lesions are often incompletely studied and, as a result, frequently present a diagnostic dilemma. Many of these incidentally identified lesions are benign. When a definitive diagnosis can be made, additional clinical imaging and work-up, with their associated costs, may be avoided.

These incidental lesions are often not resected or investigated by biopsy; hence, it is impossible accurately to determine their character or prevalence. Incidental lesions may be defined as those that are minor and relatively unimportant. In MR imaging of the knee, incidental findings are those that have no direct relationship to the patient's symptoms. This is not to suggest that these lesions have no significance; depending on the specific diagnosis of the incidental finding, follow-up may be required.

One cannot determine with certainty the prevalence of incidentally identified osseous lesions.

The lack of histologic conformation in the overwhelming majority of cases opens any review of this subject to considerable observer bias. With this caveat in mind, in this article the authors present the incidental osseous lesions that they have encountered most frequently in their personal and consultative experience during MR imaging of the knee.

This article is intended not as a complete review of the imaging findings associated with these lesions but as a summary, highlighting the MR imaging features that are most useful in suggesting a specific diagnosis.

Radiographs

Despite advances in MR imaging, the radiograph remains invaluable in evaluating bone lesions and in many cases is the most diagnostic study. Therefore, the authors strongly recommend radiographic correlation of incidentally identified lesions. Radiographs accurately predict the biologic activity of a lesion, which is reflected in the

This article was originally published in *Magnetic Resonance Imaging Clinics of North America* 15:1, February 2007.
[a] Mayo Clinic College of Medicine, Rochester, MN, USA
[b] Mayo Clinic, 4500 San Pablo Road, Jacksonville, FL 32224-3899
[c] Department of Radiology, Mayo Clinic, 4500 San Pablo Road, Jacksonville, FL 32224-3899, USA
* Corresponding author. Mayo Clinic, 4500 San Pablo Road, Jacksonville, FL 32224-3899.
E-mail address: kransdorf.mark@mayo.edu (M.J. Kransdorf).

doi:10.1016/j.rcl.2007.08.003
radiologic.theclinics.com

appearance of the lesion's margin and the type and extent of accompanying periosteal reaction. In addition, the pattern of associated matrix mineralization may be a key to the underlying histology (eg, cartilage, bone, fibro-osseous). In many cases, as in patients who have fibroxanthoma (nonossifying fibroma), osteochondroma, or enchondroma, radiographs may be virtually pathognomonic, requiring no further diagnostic imaging.

Common incidental lesions

The authors organize incidental lesions into the following broad categories: cartilaginous, fibroosseous, and degenerative. They do not address those lesions that are typically symptomatic and, as a result, likely to be directly related to the patient's clinical presentation and subsequent imaging.

Cartilaginous tumors

Cartilaginous lesions are extremely common. In surgical series, osteochondroma was the most commonly encountered benign bone tumor, representing 32% of all benign tumors in the Mayo Clinic series of 11,087 cases [1]. In the same series, enchondroma represented 12% of benign lesions [1]. These lesions are also common incidental findings, with enchondroma perhaps the most common lesion seen in adults.

Enchondroma

Enchondroma is a tumor composed of lobules of hyaline cartilage that are believed to arise from the growth plate [2]. The lesion is usually centrally located in the metaphysis of tubular bones, although great variability may be seen. Enchondromas are common and are frequent incidental

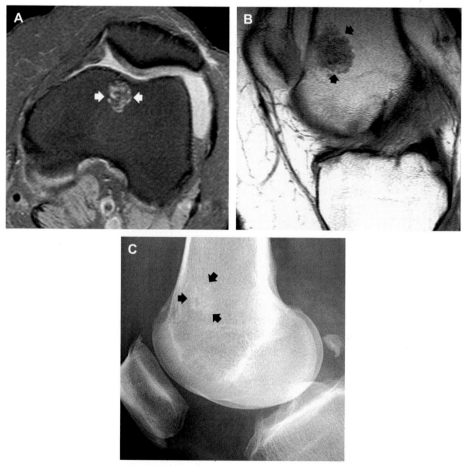

Fig. 1. Incidental enchondroma in the distal femoral metaphysis of a 68-year-old woman. (*A*) Axial fat-suppressed proton density (TR/TE; 2200/22) fast spin-echo MR image shows a well-defined eccentric lesion (*arrows*). The lesion abuts but does not scallop the cortex. (*B*) Sagittal proton density (TR/TE; 2000/20) fast spin-echo MR image shows the lobular contour to better advantage, as well as curvilinear regions of fatty marrow interdigitating between the cartilage lobules (*arrows*). (*C*) Corresponding lateral radiograph shows the subtle mineralization within the lesion (*arrows*).

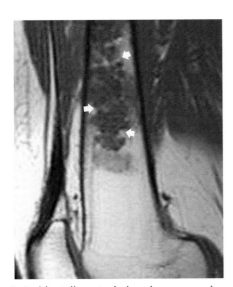

Fig. 2. Incidentally noted chondrosarcoma in a 53-year-old man. Sagittal T1-weighted (TR/TE; 491/13) spin-echo MR image shows a large cartilage tumor. The characteristic lobular contour and interdigitating marrow fat (*arrows*) are well seen. The lesion extended to the lesser trochanter, and features of malignancy were seen in the proximal aspects of the mass.

findings. In a study of 449 patients undergoing MR imaging of the knee, Murphey and colleagues [3] found incidental enchondromas in 2.9% of patients. These were most frequently encountered in the distal femur but were also seen in the proximal tibia and fibula. The lesions were located centrally in the medullary canal in 57% of patients and eccentrically in 43%.

Cohen and colleagues [4] observed a distinctive MR imaging appearance in chondroid lesions containing a matrix of hyaline cartilage. The unique pattern consisted of homogeneous high signal in a discernible lobular configuration on T2-weighted spin-echo MR images. This MRI appearance reflects the underlying high ratio of water content to mucopolysaccharide component within the hyaline cartilage [4]. On T1-weighted MR images, the lesion typically shows a signal intensity approximately equal to that of skeletal muscle, often with high-signal bands, representing medullary fat, extending between the lobules of cartilage [5]. The high signal intensity of the lesion seen on conventional T2-weighted pulse sequences tends to be somewhat reduced on fast or turbo T2-weighted images. Because the MR imaging protocols used in patients presenting for evaluation of internal derangement of the knee differ from those used when tumor is suspected, lesion morphology is increasingly important. Morphology can be especially helpful

in the diagnosis of enchondroma when it is used to identify the lobules of cartilage with intervening medullary fat (Fig. 1).

Radiographs reveal a central geographic lytic lesion, with margins varying from sclerotic to ill defined. A lobulated contour is frequently present, as is a mineralized matrix (see Fig. 1). The overlying cortex often shows endosteal scalloping or expansile remodeling, especially in the small bones of the hand, although endosteal scalloping is unusual in lesions about the knee. When lesions are not mineralized and infiltrate the medullary canal without scalloping the adjacent cortex, they may be invisible on radiographs.

Although incidental chondrosarcomas of the knee are rare (Fig. 2), the distinction between enchondroma and intramedullary chondrosarcoma of the appendicular skeleton can be difficult. MR imaging may be useful in this regard. In a review of 187 cartilage lesions, 92 enchondromas and 95 chondrosarcomas, Murphey and colleagues [6] were able to successfully differentiate these lesions in more than 90% of cases. Differentiation was based on clinical and imaging features, with the most important imaging features applicable to incidentally identified lesions being the depth and extent of endosteal scalloping (ie, greater than two thirds of cortical thickness and greater than two thirds of the lesion length).

Osteochondroma

The majority of osteochondromas are asymptomatic and discovered incidentally [7]. The lesion is believed to arise from the periphery of the physis, where an abnormal focus of metaplastic cartilage forms as a consequence of trauma or congenital perichondral deficiency [8]. Rarely, an osteochondroma may be the sequela of trauma or radiation [9]. Osteochondromas are usually classified as pedunculated or sessile (broad-based) on the basis of their morphology. Symptoms, when present, are often secondary to the size and location of the lesion or secondary fracture. Rarely, lesions may develop an overlying bursa [10]. Malignant transformation is rare. By definition, osteochondromas arise from the bone surface. The cortex of the host bone is contiguous with the stalk of the lesion, as is the medullary canal. The surface of the lesion consists of hyaline cartilage of variable thickness.

The MR imaging features of osteochondroma reflect its morphology. Both the cortex and fatty marrow of the host bone are contiguous with that of the lesion (Figs. 3, 4). The hyaline cartilage of the osteochondroma cap shows a signal intensity approximately equal to that of skeletal muscle on

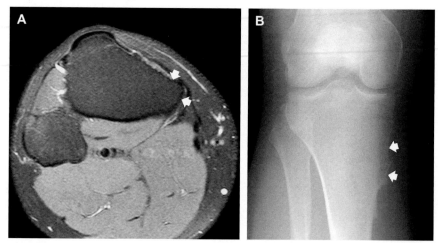

Fig. 3. Osteochondroma in the proximal tibia of a 33-year-old man. (*A*) Axial fat-suppressed proton density (TR/TE; 4000/26) fast spin-echo MR image shows a sessile osteochondroma (*arrows*) arising from proximal medial tibia. Note cortical and medullary continuity. (*B*) Corresponding anteroposterior radiograph shows the sessile osteochondroma (*arrows*).

T1-weighted images and greater than that of fat on T2-weighted images (fluid-like signal). The overlying perichondrium images as a thin peripheral zone of decreased signal intensity on T2-weighted images [11]. MR imaging also permits precise measurement of the thickness of the cartilage cap of an osteochondroma. This feature has important clinical implications, because it assists in predicting which osteochondromas are most predisposed to undergo malignant transformation to "secondary" chondrosarcoma. It is generally agreed that the risk for malignant transformation of an osteochondroma is directly related to the thickness of the cartilage cap, especially when the latter exceeds 2 or 3 cm [11,12].

Fibro-osseous lesions

Although rare specific lesions have been designated as fibro-osseous tumor of bone, this term is often used loosely for those lesions characterized by abundant fibrous or osseous tissue or both. Intraosseous lipoma is frequently associated with areas of ossification; consequently, it is also included in this broad grouping. Those lesions that are usually found incidentally include fibroxanthoma (nonossifying fibroma), benign fibrous histiocytoma, intraosseous lipoma, and bone island.

Fibroxanthoma (nonossifying fibroma)
Fibroxanthoma, nonossifying fibroma, and fibrous cortical defect are terms used to describe

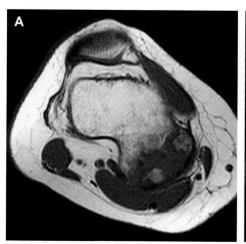

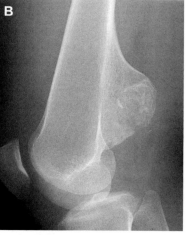

Fig. 4. Osteochondroma in the proximal tibia of a 24-year-old man. (*A*) Axial T1-weighted (TR/TE; 594/16) spin-echo MR image shows a large osteochondroma originating from the distal femoral metaphysis. (*B*) Corresponding anteroposterior radiograph shows a large, board-based osteochondroma.

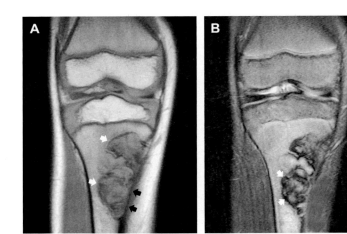
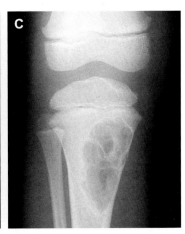

Fig. 5. Fibroxanthoma (nonossifying fibroma) in the proximal tibia of an 8-year-old boy. (*A*) Coronal T1-weighted (TR/TE; 500/14) spin-echo MR image shows a lobulated lesion (*white arrows*) in the metadiaphysis, with mild cortical scalloping and remodeling (*black arrows*). (*B*) Corresponding coronal fat-suppressed turbo T2-weighted (TR/TE; 4500/88) spin-echo MR image shows the lesion to have a low signal intensity. Note areas of markedly decreased signal intensity with "blooming," compatible with areas of hemosiderin deposition (*arrows*). (*C*) Anteroposterior radiograph of the knee shows a lobulated geographic lytic lesion with a sclerotic margin, eccentrically located in the metadiaphysis with mild cortical scalloping and remodeling, typical of a fibroxanthoma.

histologically similar lesions that occur in the metaphysis of long bones. Such lesions are quite common: Caffey [13] noted one or more of them in 36% of children studied serially. The clinical variability of the lesion has led to this confusing array of terms. Small, metaphyseal, eccentric lesions that are limited to the cortex are usually termed *fibrous cortical defects* and are likely to represent most cases described by Caffey. Persistent lesions that show interval growth and extend into the medullary cavity are usually referred to as *nonossifying fibromas* [14]. The term *fibroxanthoma* is preferred by the authors because it better reflects the underlying pathologic condition, which is composed of spindle-shaped fibroblasts, scattered giant cells, and foam (xanthoma) cells. Additionally, because these lesions may ossify and become sclerotic, use of the designation *fibroxanthoma* obviates the use of the descriptive terms *ossifying* and *nonossifying fibroma* to describe healing lesions.

The natural history of fibroxanthoma was nicely documented by Ritschl and colleagues [15] in a study of 107 lesions in 82 patients. They noted that fibroxanthomas are initially seen in the metaphysis, in the vicinity of the epiphyseal cartilage, appearing round, oval, or slightly polycyclic in shape, with well-defined nonsclerotic margins. With time, the lesion increases in size, becoming metadiaphyseal as the physis moves away from the fibroxanthoma with growth. The lesion maintains a distinct polycyclic shape, surrounded by a slightly sclerotic border. At this stage, the lesion will thin the host cortex and maintain a discrete hourglass shape.

Subsequently, the lesion will ossify, with ossification invariably starting from the diaphyseal side and progressing toward the epiphysis. Ossification continues until the fibroxanthoma is homogeneously sclerotic and then completely replaced by normal bone. The time course for this progression is variable and may range from 2.5 to 7.3 years [15]; moreover, it is unknown why some lesions progress in this orderly fashion and others continue to grow.

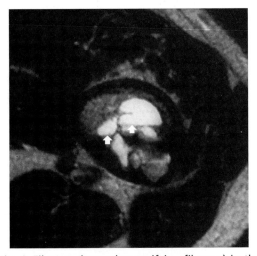

Fig. 6. Fibroxanthoma (nonossifying fibroma) in the distal femur of a 14-year-old boy. Axial T2-weighted spin-echo MR image shows multiple fluid–fluid levels (*arrows*) in a fibroxanthoma owing to secondary aneurysmal bone cyst formation.

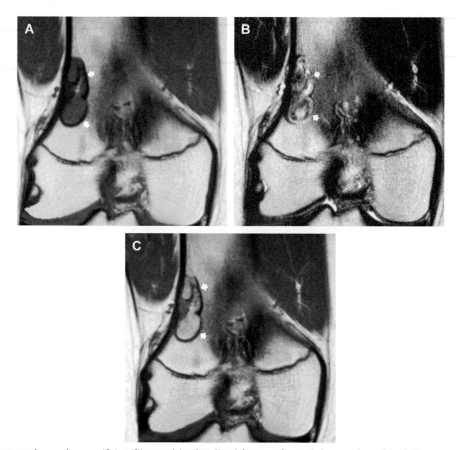

Fig. 7. Fibroxanthoma (nonossifying fibroma) in the distal femur of an adolescent boy. (*A, B*) Corresponding coronal T1-weighted (TR/TE; 450/12) spin-echo MR images preceding (*A*) and following (*B*) the administration of intravenous contrast show marked, relatively intense enhancement (*arrows*). Note typical eccentric metaphyseal location and lobulated contour. (*C*) Corresponding turbo T2-weighted (TR/TE; 4000/96) spin-echo MR image shows a heterogeneous low-to-intermediate signal intensity.

Fibroxanthomas are not uncommon incidental findings on MR imaging. Their MR imaging appearance parallels their radiographic appearance, typically demonstrating a well-defined, eccentric, scalloped, metadiaphyseal or metaphyseal geographic lesion. The MR imaging appearance is variable but most frequently demonstrates decreased signal intensity on T1- and T2-weighted spin-echo images, reflecting fibrous tissue, hemorrhage, and hemosiderin within the tumor [14,16]. Collagen and bone formation within the tumor also contribute to the finding of decreased signal intensity (Fig. 5) [16]. Less frequently, areas with a signal intensity similar to that of fat may be seen. Secondary aneurysmal bone cyst formation with fluid–fluid levels has also been reported (Fig. 6) [17]. After the administration of contrast, intense enhancement is seen in almost 80% of cases (Fig. 7), with marginal septal enhancement seen in those remaining [16]. The radiographic appearance of fibroxanthoma is virtually pathognomonic, demonstrating an eccentric, scalloped, geographic lytic lesion with a sclerotic margin in the metadiaphysis or metaphysis of long bones (see Fig. 5).

Benign fibrous histiocytoma

Benign fibrous histiocytoma of bone is histologically indistinguishable from fibroxanthoma and is separated from it only on clinical and radiologic grounds [18]. In essence, the designation of benign fibrous histiocytoma is used for fibroxanthomas with atypical radiologic or clinical manifestations (Fig. 8). O'Donnell and Saifuddin [17] reported 15 benign fibrous histiocytomas, one third of which demonstrated fluid–fluid levels on MR imaging.

Intraosseous lipoma

Although lipoma is the most common soft tissue lesion by a large margin, intraosseous lipoma is perceived as rare. Ramos and colleagues [19] noted only approximately 60 cases in their 1985 review

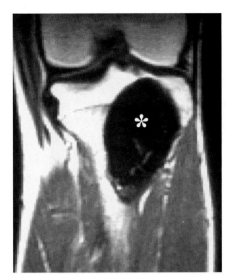

Fig. 8. Benign fibrous histiocytoma in the proximal tibia of a 19-year-old man. Coronal T1-weighted (TR/TE; 500/32) spin-echo MR image shows a well-defined lesion in the epiphysis and metaphysis of the proximal tibia (*asterisk*). Histologically, the lesion was typical of a fibroxanthoma; the marked loss of signal intensity was due to previous hemorrhage and hemosiderin deposition within the lesion. A similar appearance was seen on T2-weighted images (not shown).

of the literature. In the authors' experience, these lesions are not uncommon and are often incidental findings on examinations obtained for other reasons. Although clinical presentation is variable, pain has been reported in as many as 70% of patients [20,21].

Milgram [20] described three stages of intraosseous lipomas, which are reflected in their MR imaging appearance. Stage 1 lesions contain viable mature lipocytes, identical to those in subcutaneous fat, containing variable interspersed bony trabeculae. The osseous cortex is intact; however, mild expansile remodeling may be present. Stage 2 lesions will show areas of involution, including infarction, myxoid change, cyst formation, and often, reactive ossification. When infarction extends through the entire lesion, it is classified as a stage 3 lipoma. As a result of the central infarction, intraosseous lipoma is frequently confused with an intraosseous infarct.

On MR imaging, stage 1 lesions are well defined, with a signal intensity that mirrors that of fat on all pulse sequences. The adipose tissue within an intraosseous lipoma is devoid of hemopoietic elements and is often "fattier" than the surrounding marrow. Mild expansile remodeling is apparent in about 50% of cases (Fig. 9) [20]. Stage 2 lesions have a more complex MR imaging appearance as a result of the involutional changes, reflecting infarction, myxoid change, cyst formation, calcification, and ossification. Careful inspection, however, will reveal areas of fat within the lesion (Fig. 10). In stage 3 lesions, involutional change may completely fill the lesion, and the diagnosis may not be apparent.

Radiographic features will mirror those seen on MR imaging. Stage 1 lesions will be geographic, purely lytic lesions, with mild expansile remodeling seen in approximately 50% of cases [20]. A thin sclerotic margin is typically present in juxta-articular lesions (see Fig. 9). Stage 2 lesions will have a similar appearance and will also demonstrate

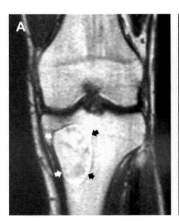
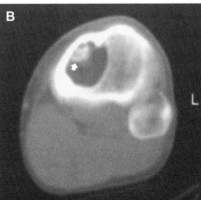
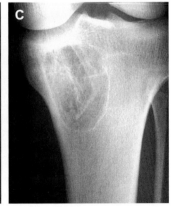

Fig. 9. Intraosseous lipoma in the proximal tibia of a 22-year-old man. (*A*) Coronal T1-weighted (TR/TE; 600/32) spin-echo MR image shows an eccentric lesion in the tibial metaphysis (*black and white arrows*), extending into the epiphysis, with a signal intensity similar to that of the adjacent marrow. (*B*) Axial CT scan shows the lesion to have an attenuation similar to that of the adjacent subcutaneous adipose tissue. Note delicate ossification within the lesion (*arrow*). (*C*) Corresponding anteroposterior radiograph shows a geographic lytic lesion with a sclerotic margin, eccentrically located in the metaphysis extending into the epiphysis.

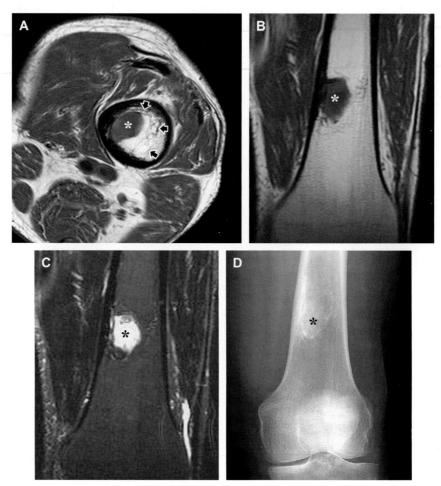

Fig. 10. Intraosseous lipoma with involutional change in the distal femur of a 72-year-old woman. (*A*) Axial T1-weighted (TR/TE; 623/17) spin-echo MR image of the distal femur shows an area of cyst formation (*asterisk*) within the lesion. Portions of the lesion are well delineated by marginal sclerosis (*arrows*), whereas other areas are poorly defined. (*B, C*) Corresponding coronal T1-weighted (TR/TE; 620/17) (*B*) spin-echo and short-tau inversion recovery (TR/TE/TI; 7870/86/160) (*C*) MR images show the involutional cyst (*asterisk*), although the margins are incompletely visualized. (*D*) Anteroposterior radiograph of the distal femur shows a thin mineralized margin around the cyst (*asterisk*). Portions of the mineralized margin around the lesion are also visualized.

areas of mineralization (see Fig. 10). Stage 3 lesions demonstrate greater involutional change with reactive ossification, frequently with associated peripherally mineralized cyst formation [10,20]. The cysts within lipomas may become hemorrhagic, with subsequent alterations in the MR signal intensity [22].

Recently, Wada and Lambert [23] reported a case of a simple bone cyst treated with intralesional corticosteroids, and subsequently with intralesional ethanol, that developed a rind of fat at the periphery of the lesion, mimicking an intraosseous lipoma with involutional change. It is not clear whether such a process could occur spontaneously; however, it does raise an interesting question as to the true nature of intraosseous lipomas.

Bone island

A bone island, also termed enostosis, is a focal intraosseous mass of compact lamellar bone with Haversian systems, which blends into the surrounding cancellous bone [24]. Most lesions are between 2 mm and 2 cm in size and are located in the juxta-articular regions of long bones, oriented along the long axis of the bone. It is difficult to determine the prevalence of bone islands; however, they are extremely common and seen with equal frequency in men and women [10].

MR imaging reflects the lesion's morphology. Because the lesion simulates cortical bone histologically, the MR imaging appearance will reflect the signal intensity of cortical bone, with a complete loss of signal on all pulse sequences [25]. The

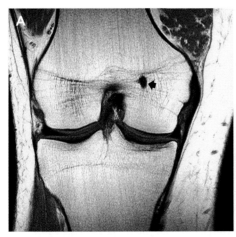
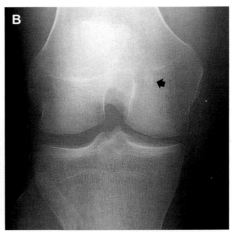

Fig. 11. Bone island (enostosis) in the medial femoral epiphysis in a 22-year-old man. (*A*) Coronal weighted (TR/TE; 704/14) spin-echo MR image of the distal femur shows an oval focus of decreased signal intensity (*arrow*). The lesion blends into the surrounding cancellous bone, yielding a spiculated margin. (*B*) Anteroposterior radiograph of the distal femur shows a subtle bone island (*arrow*) corresponding to the lesion seen on MR imaging.

fusion of the mass with the surrounding cancellous bone will give rise to a "paint-brush" or "spiculated" margin (Fig. 11) [24]. Although bone islands are usually small, "giant" bone islands have been described (Fig. 12). It has been the authors' experience that these large lesions may be somewhat heterogeneous on MR imaging. Radiographs will show a single or multiple, homogeneously dense, ovoid, round, or oblong focus of sclerosis with a spiculated margin (see Fig. 11) [26].

Degenerative lesions

Degenerative joint disease is the most commonly encountered articular disorder. The imaging manifestations of degenerative arthritis usually allow a satisfactory diagnosis; however, when osteoarthritic cysts become the dominant radiologic feature, the underlying diagnosis may be less apparent.

Osteoarthritic cyst

The most common intraosseous lesion identified during MR imaging evaluation of the knee in older adults is the subchondral degenerative cyst. Also termed synovial cyst, subchondral cyst, degenerative cyst, subarticular pseudocyst, and geode, these lesions are a prominent finding in patients who have osteoarthritis [27]. Although the designation of "cyst" is used to describe this lesion, this term is inaccurate, in that it implies a fluid-filled, epithelial-lined cavity [27]. Degenerative subchondral cysts are not lined by epithelium, nor are they uniformly fluid filled. The term geode is used in geology to describe a hollow, usually spheroidal rock with crystals lining the inside wall [27].

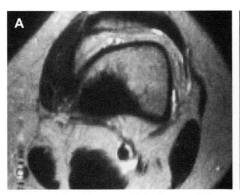
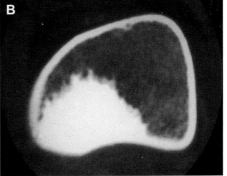

Fig. 12. Giant bone island (enostosis) in the distal femur. (*A*) Axial T2-weighted spin-echo MR image of the distal femur shows a large mass with decreased signal intensity, similar to that of cortical bone, and spiculated margins with the adjacent marrow. T1-weighted image (not shown) had a similar appearance. (*B*) Corresponding noncontrast CT scan shows the spiculated margin to better advantage.

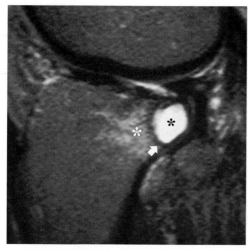

Fig. 13. Subchondral cyst in the proximal tibia. Sagittal T2-weighted spin-echo MR image of the proximal tibia shows a small, well-defined, fluid-like mass, adjacent to the articular surface (*black asterisk*). Note subtle adjacent edema-like signal (*white asterisk*) and marginal sclerosis (*arrow*).

Two theories exist regarding the pathogenesis of subchondral cysts in osteoarthritis. One suggests that the mechanism is elevated intra-articular pressure, with intrusion of synovial fluid through the cartilage and subsequent subchondral cyst formation [28]. The other surmises that the impaction of apposing bony surfaces results in fracture and vascular insufficiency of the subchondral bone, leading to cystic necrosis [29]. Regardless of whether one or both of these mechanisms is at play, cystic spaces develop in the subchondral bone [27,30].

Subchondral cysts may also develop following injury. Although the mechanism of posttraumatic subchondral cyst formation is not known, it is reasonable to suspect that these same processes are at play. Posttraumatic cysts have a similar appearance to degenerative cysts, although they are typically larger [27]. Similar to degenerative subchondral cysts, posttraumatic cysts may communicate with the joint.

Cysts are often multiple and variable in size; they are typically well marginated with a thin sclerotic margin and are associated with joint space narrowing, osteophyte formation, and subchondral sclerosis. In cases with prominent features of osteoarthritis, the diagnosis is usually made without difficulty. MR imaging has been shown to be markedly more sensitive in detecting subchondral cysts [31,32]. The MR imaging appearance of these common lesions reflects their pathophysiology: a focal, round-to-oval, subchondral cyst–like lesion, with an intermediate to high signal intensity on fluid-sensitive sequences. A thin sclerotic margin is often appreciated as a rind of decreased signal intensity at the periphery of the lesion. The authors often note associated surrounding nonspecific edema-like signal (Fig. 13). Single or large (greater than 2 cm) cysts are unusual, and they are frequently mistaken for more sinister processes (Fig. 14).

Radiographically, these lesions are well defined with a sclerotic margin that may—or, more typically

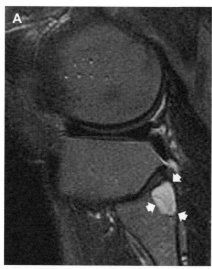
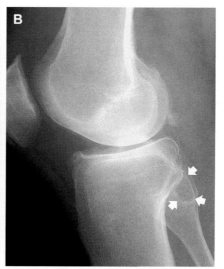

Fig. 14. Subchondral cyst in the proximal fibula. (*A*) Sagittal T2-weighted (TR/TE; 2300/80) spin-echo MR image of the proximal fibula shows a focal high-signal intensity eccentric mass (*arrows*), immediately adjacent to the articular surface. The absence of significant associated degenerative arthritis suggested the possible diagnosis of a giant cell tumor. (*B*) Corresponding lateral radiograph shows the lesion to have a well-defined sclerotic margin (*arrows*), in keeping with a degenerative subchondral cyst.

in the authors' experience, may not—communicate with the joint. Lesions are often found adjacent to the cruciate ligament attachments [33]. An adjacent soft tissue ganglion may be present, and gas may be present within either component. Schajowicz and colleagues [34] noted that 15% of cases in their series resulted from penetration of a soft tissue ganglion into the underlying bone, whereas the remaining cases resulted from altered mechanical stresses leading to vascular disturbances, foci of bone necrosis, with subsequent healing.

Intraosseous ganglion

Intraosseous ganglia are solitary, unilocular or multilocular lesions found at or near the ends of long bones in the subchondral region [34]. Typically occurring in middle-aged adults who present with mild, localized pain, the lesion is similar to a soft tissue ganglion [35,36]. The pathogenesis of intraosseous ganglia is unclear, and there is debate as to whether this entity may be differentiated from degenerative subchondral or posttraumatic cysts. Although they are not histologically unique, intraosseous ganglia are characterized by fibroblastic proliferation and mucoid degeneration. Those who use this designation typically reserve it for intraosseous lesions resembling subchondral cysts in patients who have little or no degenerative arthritis in the adjacent articulation.

Summary

Incidental osseous lesions are commonly identified in patients undergoing MR imaging of the knee. Although a wide spectrum of lesions may be seen, the most common lesions may often be successfully diagnosed on the basis of their MR imaging findings and correlating radiographs.

References

[1] Unni KK. Dahlin's bone tumors: general aspects and data on 11,087 cases. 5th edition. Philadelphia: Lippincott-Raven; 1996. p. 1–9.

[2] Milgram JW. The origins of osteochondromas and enchondromas. A histopathologic study. Clin Orthop Relat Res 1983;174:264–84.

[3] Murphey MD, Walden MJ, Vidal JA. Incidental enchondromas of the knee [abstract]. Skeletal Radiol 2007;36:359.

[4] Cohen EK, Kressel HY, Frank TS, et al. Hyaline cartilage–origin bone and soft tissue neoplasms: MR appearance and histologic correlation. Radiology 1988;167:477–81.

[5] Aoki J, Sone S, Fujioka F, et al. MR of enchondroma and chondrosarcoma: rings and arcs of Gd-DTPA enhancement. J Comput Assist Tomogr 1991;15:1011–6.

[6] Murphey MD, Walker EA, Wilson AJ, et al. From the archives of the AFIP: imaging of primary chondrosarcoma: radiologic–pathologic correlation. Radiographics 2003;23:1245–78.

[7] Woertler K. Benign bone tumors and tumor-like lesions: value of cross-sectional imaging. Eur Radiol 2003;13:1820–35.

[8] D'Ambrosia R, Ferguson AB. The formation of osteochondroma by epiphyseal cartilage transplantation. Clin Orthop Relat Res 1968;61:103–15.

[9] Libshitz HI, Cohen MA. Radiation-induced osteochondromas. Radiology 1982;142:643–7.

[10] Resnick D, Kyriakos M, Greenway GD. Tumor and tumor-like lesions of bone: imaging of specific lesions. In: Resnick D, editor. Diagnosis of bone and joint disorders. 4th edition. Philadelphia: W.B. Saunders; 2002. p. 3763–4128.

[11] Lee JK, Yao L, Wirth CR. MR imaging of solitary osteochondromas: report of eight cases. AJR Am J Roentgenol 1987;149:557–60.

[12] Hudson TM, Springfield DS, Spanier SS, et al. Benign exostoses and exostotic chondrosarcomas: evaluation of cartilage thickness by CT. Radiology 1984;151:595–9.

[13] Caffey J. On fibrous defects in cortical walls of growing tubular bones. Adv Pediatr 1955;7:13–51.

[14] Kransdorf MJ, Utz JA, Gilkey FW, et al. MR appearance of fibroxanthoma. J Comput Assist Tomogr 1989;12:612–5.

[15] Ritschl P, Karnel F, Hajek P. Fibrous metaphyseal defects—determination of their origin and natural history using a radiomorphological study. Skeletal Radiol 1988;17:8–15.

[16] Jee W, Choe B, Kang H, et al. Nonossifying fibroma: characteristics at MR imaging with pathologic correlation. Radiology 1998;209:197–202.

[17] O'Donnell P, Saifuddin A. The prevalence and diagnostic significance of fluid–fluid levels in focal lesions of bone. Skeletal Radiol 2004;33:330–6.

[18] Kyriakos M. Benign fibrous histiocytoma of bone. In: Christopher DM, Unni KK, Mertens F, editors. WHO classification of tumors. Pathology and genetics: tumors of soft tissue and bone. Lyon (France): IARC Press; 2002. p. 292–3.

[19] Ramos A, Castello J, Sartoris DJ, et al. Osseous lipoma: CT appearance. AJR Am J Roentgenol 1985;157:615–9.

[20] Milgram JW. Intraosseous lipomas. A clinicopathologic study of 66 cases. Clin Orthop Relat Res 1988;231:277–302.

[21] Campbell RSD, Grainger AJ, Mangham DC, et al. Intraosseous lipoma: report of 35 new cases and a review of the literature. Skeletal Radiol 2003; 32:209–22.

[22] Kwak HS, Lee KB, Lee SY, et al. MR findings of calcaneal intraosseous lipoma with hemorrhage. AJR Am J Roentgenol 2005;185:1378–9.

[23] Wada R, Lambert RGW. Deposition of intraosseous fat in a degenerating simple bone cyst. Skeletal Radiol 2005;43:415–8.

[24] Mirra JM. Bone tumors: clinical, radiologic and pathologic correlations. Philadelphia: Lea & Febiger; 1989. p. 143–438.

[25] Cerase A, Priolo F. Skeletal benign bone-forming lesions. Eur J Radiol 1998;27:S91–7.

[26] Greenspan A, Steiner G, Knutzon R. Bone island (enostosis): clinical significance and radiologic and pathologic correlations. Skeletal Radiol 1991;20:85–90.

[27] Resnick D. Degenerative disease of extraspinal locations. In: Resnick D, editor. Diagnosis of bone and joint disorders. 4th edition. Philadelphia: W.B. Saunders Company; 2002. p. 1271–381.

[28] Freund E. The pathological significance of intra-articular pressure. Edinburgh Med J 1940;47:192–203.

[29] Rhaney K, Lamb DW. The cysts of osteoarthritis of the hip: a radiologic and pathologic study. J Bone Joint Surg Br 1955;37:663–75.

[30] Resnick D, Niwayama G, Coutts RD. Subchondral cysts (geodes) in arthritic disorders: pathologic and radiographic appearance of the hip joint. AJR Am J Roentgenol 1977;128:799–806.

[31] Burk DL, Kanal E, Brunberg JA, et al. 1.5-T surface-coil MRI of the knee. AJR Am J Roentgenol 1986;147:293–300.

[32] Poleksic L, Zdravkovic D, Jablanovic D, et al. Magnetic resonance imaging of bone destruction in rheumatoid arthritis: comparison with radiography. Skeletal Radiol 1993; 22:577–80.

[33] Stacy GS, Heck RK, Peabody TD, et al. Neoplastic and tumorlike lesions detected on MR imaging of the knee in patients with suspected internal derangement: part 1, intraosseous entities. AJR Am J Roentgenol 2002;178:589–94.

[34] Schajowicz F, Clavel Sainz M, Slullitel JA. Juxta-articular bone cysts (intra-osseous ganglia): a clinicopathological study of eighty-eight cases. J Bone Joint Surg Br 1979;61:107–16.

[35] Magee TH, Rowedder AM, Degnan GG. Intraosseous ganglia of the wrist. Radiology 1995;195: 517–20.

[36] Pope TL, Fechner RE, Keats TE. Intra-osseous ganglion. Skeletal Radiol 1989;18:185–8.

RADIOLOGIC CLINICS OF NORTH AMERICA

Radiol Clin N Am 45 (2007) 955–968

Osseous and Myotendinous Injuries About the Knee

Thomas H. Berquist, MD, FACR[a,b,*]

- Osseous injuries
  - *Bone bruise or marrow edema pattern*
  - *Stress and insufficiency fractures*
  - *Tibial plateau fractures*
  - *Segond and reverse Segond fractures*
  - *Fibular head avulsion fractures*
  - *Fractures in children*
  - *Osteochondral lesions*
  - *Spontaneous osteonecrosis of the knee*
- Myotendinous injuries
  - *Quadriceps injuries*
  - *Patellar tendon injuries*
  - *Patellar retinacular tears*
  - *Gastrocnemius, soleus, and plantaris injuries*
  - *Popliteus muscle injuries*
  - *Iliotibial band syndrome*
  - *Other myotendinous injuries*
- References

Osseous injuries

Osseous injuries may be articular, extra-articular, or physeal, and may be related to direct trauma, avulsion forces, or chronic microtrauma [1–3]. Displaced fractures can be diagnosed easily on radiographs; however, multiple, subtle osseous or osteochondral lesions may not be defined radiographically. In addition, subtle findings on MR images, such as bone bruises, can be useful for evaluating the mechanism and extent of bone and soft-tissue involvement [4]. MR imaging is also a valuable technique for the detection and follow-up evaluation of children with physeal injuries [5,6]. Table 1 summarizes osseous and osteochondral injuries about the knee, and optimal imaging approaches.

Bone bruise or marrow edema pattern

Bone bruises or marrow edema may be identified with numerous conditions, including trauma, infection, and osteoporosis [4,7–9]. Bone bruises related to trauma may be caused by a direct blow, articular compression forces, or avulsion injuries [4]. The extent of marrow edema tends to be more dramatic with compression or direct trauma, compared with avulsion injuries [8]. Typically, bone bruises are not visible on radiographs. However, these injuries are detected easily on MR images using T1-weighted sequences and either short T1 inversion recovery (STIR) or fat-suppressed T2-weighted sequences (Fig. 1) [1,7]. Specific edema patterns are also useful in predicting the mechanism of injury and the associated ligament, tendon, or meniscal involvement [4]. Five classic patterns have been described.

Patients who have pivot shift injuries typically have bone contusions involving the posterior lateral tibial plateau and midlateral femoral condyle. The posterior margin of the medial tibial plateau may be involved as well. Associated injuries include the anterior cruciate ligament, the posterior

This article was originally published in *Magnetic Resonance Imaging Clinics of North America* 15:1, February 2007.

[a] Department of Diagnostic Radiology, Mayo Clinic College of Medicine, Rochester, MN 55901, USA

[b] Department of Diagnostic Radiology, E2 Mayo Clinic Jacksonville, 4500 San Pablo Road, Jacksonville, FL 32224, USA

* Department of Diagnostic Radiology, E2 Mayo Clinic Jacksonville, 4500 San Pablo Road, Jacksonville, FL 32224.

E-mail address: berquist.thomas@mayo.edu

Table 1: Subtle osteochondral injuries about the knee

Injury	Imaging approaches	Comments
Bone bruise	Radiographs, then MR imaging	Assess ligaments, menisci, other soft-tissue injuries
Stress and insufficiency fractures	Radiographs, then MR imaging	Confirm fracture, exclude other pathology
Physeal fractures	Radiographs, then MR imaging	Detect, exclude growth plate closure
Tibial spine fractures	Radiographs, then MR imaging	Classify, exclude ACL and other injuries
Avulsion fractures	Radiographs, then MR imaging or CT	Detect, exclude soft-tissue injuries
Segond fractures	Radiographs, then MR imaging	Assess ACL, menisci, and other soft-tissue injuries
Reverse Segond fractures	Radiographs, then MR imaging	Assess PCL, menisci, and other soft-tissue injuries
Tibial plateau fractures	Radiographs, then MR imaging or CT	Assess articular deformity and separation, and soft-tissue and meniscal injuries
Fibular head avulsion fractures	Radiographs, then MR imaging	Assess posterolateral corner injury and PCL injury
Osteochondritis dissecans	Radiographs, then MR imaging	Confirm and classify

Abbreviations: ACL, anterior cruciate ligament; PCL, posterior cruciate ligament.

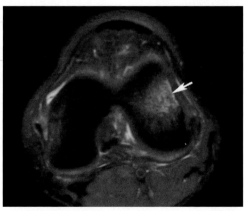

Fig. 1. Fat-suppressed fast spin-echo T2-weighted image demonstrates a bone bruise in the lateral femoral condyle (*arrow*).

Patients who have hyperextension of the knee present with kissing contusions of the anterior tibia and the adjacent anterior distal femur. Hyperextension injuries also may involve cruciate ligaments, the menisci, and, if severe enough, the posterior capsule and neurovascular structures posterior to the knee.

Clipping injuries, classically seen in football, result in prominent lateral femoral condyle edema and a smaller area of contusion in the medial femoral condyle. Medial collateral ligament injuries are common (Fig. 2). When more severe valgus force is applied, the anterior cruciate ligament and medial meniscus may be torn as well (O'Donoghue's triad).

Finally, lateral patellar dislocations lead to bone bruises or contusions involving the medial patellar articular surface and the anterior lateral femoral condyle. The medial retinaculum, the medial patellofemoral ligament, and the medial patellotibial ligament all may be disrupted with this injury pattern [4].

Stress and insufficiency fractures

Insufficiency fractures occur when normal stress or muscle tension acts on bone, with abnormal elastic resistance. These fractures commonly occur in the elderly population or in debilitated patients who have reduced bone stock (Fig. 3). Stress fractures or stress reactions result from repetitive stresses, less than those required to produce a complete fracture in normal bone.

Most stress fractures in the knee are related to running, jumping, or hurdling [2,10]. Stress fractures about the knee are common and may involve the proximal tibia, fibula, distal femur, patella, or fabella. Seventy-five per cent of exertional leg pain and stress fractures involve the tibia [10]. The proximal tibia is the most common site for stress fractures in the knee [2].

capsule, the arcuate ligament, and the posterior horn of the medial or lateral meniscus. The medial collateral ligament may be disrupted also.

A dashboard injury or direct trauma to the anterior tibia results in marrow edema in the anterior tibia. The posterior cruciate ligament and the posterior capsule may be torn with this injury pattern.

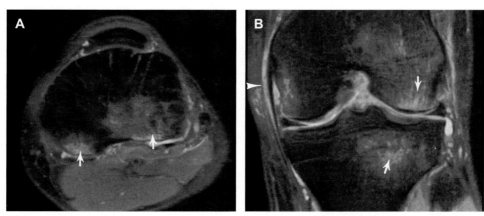

Fig. 2. Football injury associated with valgus and rotational forces. Axial (*A*) and coronal (*B*) fat-suppressed fast spin-echo T2-weighted images demonstrate posterior tibial bone bruises (*arrows in A*) with lateral femoral and tibial bruises (*arrows in B*) caused by valgus stress. The increased signal intensity in the medial collateral ligament (*arrowhead*) is caused by ligament sprain. The anterior cruciate ligament is also torn.

Radiographs are insensitive during the early phases of these injuries. Although radionuclide scans are sensitive during the early phases, they are less specific than MR imaging. Considering the numerous causes of bone pain about the knee, it is important to employ an imaging modality that is both sensitive and specific, so that more serious conditions, such as neoplasm, are not overlooked [1,2,10–12]. MR imaging has become the technique of choice for evaluating stress injuries. Injuries can be detected early, before an actual fracture line develops. Fredericson and colleagues [12] developed a system based on periosteal and marrow involvement on T1- and T2-weighted or STIR MR images. Grade 1 lesions demonstrate periosteal edema on T2-weighted or STIR images with normal marrow signal intensity. Grade 2 lesions demonstrate

periosteal edema and marrow edema on T2 or STIR sequences, with little change on T1-weighted sequences. Grade 3 injuries demonstrate more significant periosteal changes, and marrow signal is abnormal on T1- and T2-weighted or STIR sequences. Grade 4 injuries demonstrate a clear fracture line (Fig. 4). Some investigators have also included Grade 0 for normal [1,10,12]. Usually, contrast enhancement is not necessary and is not included in the grading system.

Tibial plateau fractures

Subtle tibial plateau fractures are overlooked easily on radiographs. The only finding may be a lipohemarthrosis, which can be detected on the cross-table lateral radiograph. Displaced tibial plateau fractures are detected easily on radiographs.

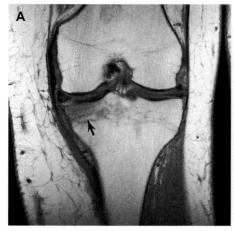
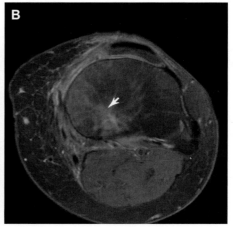

Fig. 3. Tibial insufficiency fracture. Coronal T1- (*A*) and axial fat-suppressed fast spin-echo T2- (*B*) weighted images demonstrate abnormal signal intensity in the proximal medial tibia (*black and white arrows*). Meniscal degeneration is also shown.

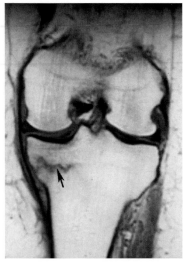

Fig. 4. Tibial stress fracture. Coronal T1-weighted image demonstrates a grade 4 stress fracture with a fracture line (*arrow*) in the medial tibia.

However, further imaging with CT or MR imaging is required to evaluate fragment position and associated soft-tissue injuries. CT is adequate for the evaluation of fracture position, articular step-off, and separation of fragments. MR imaging, especially with subtle fractures, can assess the bony injury and associated ligament and meniscal injury more easily (Fig. 5) [2,13]. Holt and colleagues [13], reviewed the MR features of tibial plateau fractures and found that its ability to detect occult injuries was superior to other modalities. In addition, the fractures were reclassified in 48% of patients and management was altered in 19% of cases.

Segond and reverse Segond fractures

The Segond fracture and its rare counterpart, the reverse Segond fracture, appear innocuous on radiographs. The first is a small, avulsion fracture proximal and posterior to the insertion of the iliotibial band on Gerdy's tubercle. This injury may be associated with several mechanisms. The avulsion may occur with internal rotation and the knee flexed, or with internal rotation and varus stress. The fracture is caused by avulsion of the meniscotibial portion of the middle third of the lateral capsular ligament, with possible associated fractures of the fibular head or Gerdy's tubercle [2,14]. In the case of severe varus stress, such as in a motor vehicle accident, the entire lateral ligament complex may be disrupted [14]. Segond fractures have a high incidence of anterior cruciate ligament tears and meniscal injury. MR imaging is ideal for the detection of osseous, meniscal, and ligament injuries (Fig. 6) [1,2,14].

The reverse Segond fracture, much less common, is a medial avulsion of the deep medial collateral ligament attachment on the tibia. The mechanism of injury is felt to be valgus stress with external rotation [15] and is associated with disruption of the posterior cruciate ligament and peripheral medial meniscus tears. Again, when this avulsion is detected on radiographs, MR imaging should be performed to evaluate the associated ligament and meniscal injuries [1,15].

Fibular head avulsion fractures

Avulsion of the styloid of the fibular head can be detected on the anteroposterior, lateral, or internal oblique radiographs. On the anteroposterior view, the fragment may mimic a Segond fracture [16]. This injury is termed the "arcuate sign" because it indicates avulsion of the arcuate complex (fabellofibular, popliteofibular, and arcuate) ligaments. This injury results in posterior lateral instability. The mechanism of injury is a direct blow to the anterior medial tibia with the knee in extension [16]. MR imaging is important for evaluating these patients because all reported cases have had associated

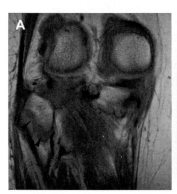
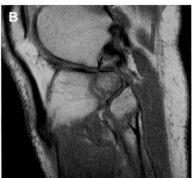
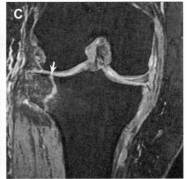

Fig. 5. Lateral tibial plateau and fibular fractures. Coronal (*A*) and sagittal (*B*) T1-weighted and coronal dual-echo in steady state (DESS) (*C*) images demonstrate a fibular fracture and lateral tibial plateau fracture with slight separation and articular step-off. Tibial plateau fracture (*arrows; B, C*), and fibular fracture (*arrowheads; A, B*).

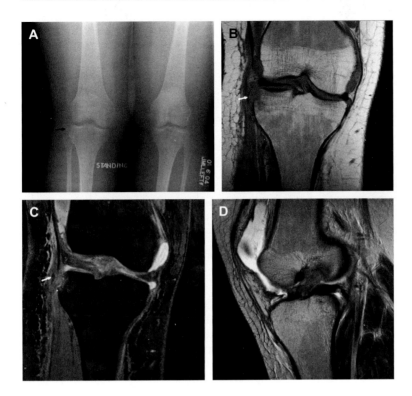

Fig. 6. Segond fracture. (*A*) Anteroposterior radiograph of the knees demonstrates a flake fracture from the proximal tibia laterally (*arrow*). Coronal T1-weighted (*B*), DESS (*C*), and sagittal proton density (*D*) images demonstrate the fracture (*arrows*), a large joint effusion, and anterior cruciate ligament tear.

posterior cruciate ligament tears. No anterior cruciate ligament tears have been reported. Also, MR images may demonstrate edema of the fibular head, although less commonly than a frank avulsion; this finding should also make one consider arcuate ligament complex injury [16].

Other locations of avulsion fractures about the knee include the posterior medial tibia because of semimembranosus tendon avulsion, and the lateral femoral condyle at the popliteus insertion [14].

Fractures in children

Fractures in children deserve a separate discussion. Physeal fractures are classified using the Salter-Harris system. Fractures of the distal femoral growth plate account for 7% of all physeal injuries. Proximal tibial growth plate fractures are less common and account for only 3% of all physeal fractures [17]. Salter-Harris II fractures occur most commonly in the femur and tibia. Most fractures are caused by hyperextension, which may lead to injury of the posterior neurovascular structures. Angular deformity and leg length discrepancy may result, especially with Salter-Harris III to V fractures [3,6,17].

Tibial eminence (spine) fractures may occur in adults, but are much more common in children [17,18]. This injury occurs most often between the ages of 8 and 14. Again, hyperextension is the most common mechanism of injury. Myers and

McKeever [19] categorized tibial eminence fractures into three types, based on the position of the fragments. Type I fractures are nondisplaced and account for 16% of injuries; type II factures are elevated anteriorly (39% of fractures); and type III fractures are displaced (45% of fractures). Type I and II fractures can be treated with closed reduction, whereas type III fractures require surgical intervention (Fig. 7) [17].

Tibial tuberosity fractures are divided into three categories as well. Type I fractures are small, avulsed fragments and account for 39% of tuberosity fractures (Fig. 8); type II fractures result in anterior hinging of the entire tuberosity (18%); and type III fractures extend into the tibial articular surface [19]. Type I fractures may be treated with cast immobilization. Type II and III fractures require reduction, with cancellous bone screws [17,19].

Radiographs can be used to define most of these injuries, especially if the fracture is displaced. However, MR imaging may be required to detect subtle fractures (see Figs. 7 and 8) during the healing process. This imaging is important especially with growth plate fractures [1–3,6,17]. Multiplanar MR imaging with T2-weighted or STIR sequences is useful for evaluating physeal fractures and assessing bone bars that may lead to angular deformity or growth arrest. MR imaging can identify and measure the degree of bony bar formation, which permits the orthopedic surgeon to make appropriate

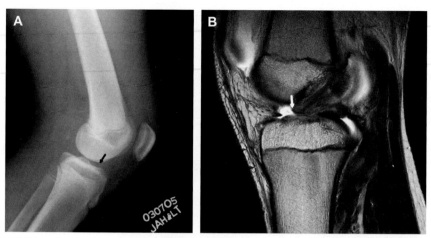

Fig. 7. Type III tibial eminence fracture. Lateral radiograph (*A*) and T2-weighted sagittal MR image (*B*) demonstrate a subtle eminence avulsion (*black and white arrows*).

decisions regarding operative intervention (Fig. 9). Physeal arrest or bone bars measuring less that 25% of the growth plate can be resected with good results. Surgical correction does not provide good results if more that 40% of the growth plate is involved [3].

Osteochondral lesions

Osteochondral lesions in the knee may be acute or chronic, and include conditions such as osteochondritis dissecans (OCD) [20]. Acute lesions result from impaction, or rotational or shearing forces. The fracture may involve only cartilage, or cartilage and underlying bone. The fracture line is parallel to the joint line, unlike more conventional fractures that enter the joint vertically or obliquely. Fractures may be impacted, elevated partially or displaced, or displaced completely and free in the joint [20,21].

OCD may have a similar appearance, although its presentation is more insidious or chronic in nature.

Classically, OCD involves the lateral aspect of the medial femoral condyle in the knee. However, the patella and other sites may be involved as well. When imaging osteochondral lesions, radiographs may be useful, but detection and appropriate classification are accomplished more effectively with MR imaging using T1- and T2-weighted or STIR sequences. The axial and sagittal planes are most useful for femoral lesions, but all image planes, including the coronal, should be evaluated carefully [1,22]. Classification of these lesions is important for management decisions (Fig. 10). Lesions that are minimal (softening, fibrillation, or fissuring) show abnormal signal intensity without elevation or separation. These lesions may be treated with non–weight bearing activities for 6 to 12 weeks. Partially or completely displaced lesions that remain in the native bed may be reattached during arthroscopy. Lesions that are displaced and free in the joint are removed. Large bone defects

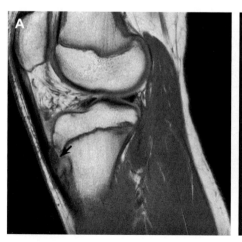

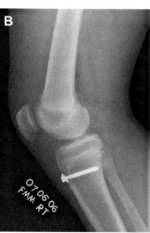

Fig. 8. Type I tibial tuberosity avulsion. Sagittal T1-weighted image (*A*) demonstrates a tibial tuberosity avulsion (*arrow*). The fragment was reduced with a cancellous screw (*B*).

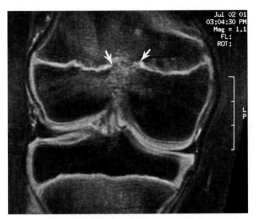

Fig. 9. Coronal STIR image demonstrates a bone bar (*arrows*) involving about 10% of the physis.

can be drilled or transplanted with autologous cartilage, but the latter is still under evaluation [20].

DeSmet and colleagues [21] evaluated MR signs of unstable lesions. These findings included a high signal intensity line between the native bone and the osteochondral fragment (72%), focal defects (31%), articular fracture (25%), and adjacent subchondral cysts (22%). The first finding was the most accurate, compared with arthroscopic findings (Fig. 11).

Spontaneous osteonecrosis of the knee

Spontaneous osteonecrosis of the knee was considered classically a condition of vascular insufficiency, leading to bone infarction of the weight-bearing surface of the femoral condyle (Fig. 12). The condition was seen in older adults, unlike OCD, which commonly occurs in adolescents. The condition almost always was unilateral and involved most commonly the medial femoral condyle (Fig. 13) [23].

In more recent years, changes seen with spontaneous osteonecrosis have been questioned because of similarities to subchondral fractures in the femoral head. A growing base of knowledge in the literature suggests that a subchondral insufficiency fracture leads to focal osteonecrosis [24,25]. Similar features have been described in the medial tibial plateau as well [25].

Myotendinous injuries

Muscle and tendon injuries about the knee may occur alone or in association with more significant osseous and ligament injuries. Muscle and tendon injuries may be related to direct trauma (muscle contusion) or to indirect trauma with overextension. Indirect injuries may result in partial or complete disruption, and are classified as strains. Avulsion injuries may also occur. Tendon and

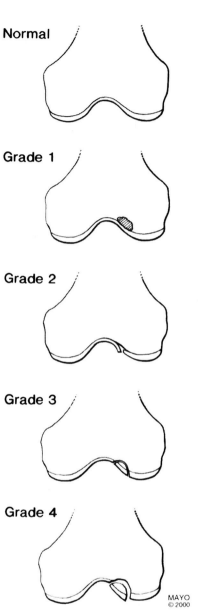

Fig. 10. MR features of OCD. Normal articular cartilage is Grade 0. Grade 1 shows abnormal signal intensity with cartilage intact. Grade 2 lesions demonstrate a linear cleft in the articular cartilage. Grade 3 lesions have abnormal signal intensity surrounding the lesion, and Grade 4 lesions are displaced. (*Courtesy of* the Mayo Foundation for Medical Education and Research; used with permission. All rights reserved.)

muscle strains are categorized as first degree, when only a few fibers are torn; second degree, when about 50% of fibers are torn; and third degree, when there is a complete tear [1,26,27]. Hematomas commonly form with higher-grade injuries. Depending on the location, more aggressive

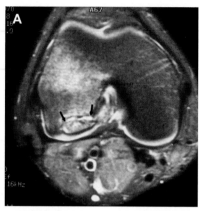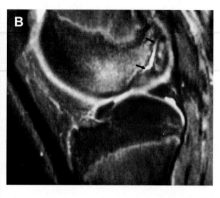

Fig. 11. Grade 4 OCD. Axial (*A*) and sagittal (*B*) T2-weighted images demonstrate fluid signal intensity (*arrows*) between the osteochondral lesion and the femur. Slight displacement of the fragment is also shown.

therapy, with evacuation of the hematoma, may be required [1,26].

Avulsion fractures may be evident on radiographs but MR imaging is the technique of choice for detection and classification of muscle and tendon injuries. Imaging should be performed in the two most appropriate planes (axial plus coronal, sagittal, or oblique), using T2-weighted or STIR sequences to identify and grade the level of injury. Other associated injuries can be detected also [1,26–28].

Quadriceps injuries

Injury to the quadriceps mechanism (rectus femoris, vastus medialis, vastus intermedius, vastus lateralis, and quadriceps tendon) may be the result of acute trauma caused by rapid deceleration, such as running when the foot is planted, or it may be caused by chronic microtrauma. In elderly patients or patients who have gout, diabetes, connective tissue diseases, or other systemic conditions, minor

trauma may result in quadriceps injury [1,26,29]. Most injuries occur distally at, or near, the patellar attachment (Fig. 14) [29,30]. Patients who have first- or second-degree strains still can extend the knee. Third-degree strains (complete tear) result in an inability to extend the knee (see Fig. 14) and require surgical repair [1,29]. MR imaging in the axial and sagittal planes can grade the level of injury accurately [1].

Patellar tendon injuries

Patellar tendon injuries may be caused by chronic overuse ("jumper's knee," tendonosis, or tendinitis) or more acute injuries with partial or complete tendon tears [1,2,29,31–35]. Most injuries are caused by chronic microtrauma, resulting in tendinitis or tendonosis and partial tears at the inferior pole of the patella. These injuries are seen commonly in athletes involved in jumping; hence, the term jumper's knee [31,32,34]. Activities such as basketball, tennis, soccer, and track are associated most

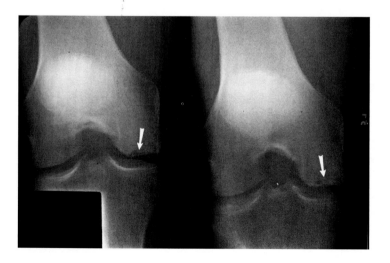

Fig. 12. Notch views of the knee demonstrates osteochondral collapse (*arrows*) of the weight-bearing surface of the medial femoral condyle. (*From* Kelley EA, Berquist TH. The knee. In: Berquist TH, editor. MRI of the musculoskeletal system. 5th edition. Philadelphia: Lipincott-Williams and Wilkins; 2006. p. 303–429; with permission.)

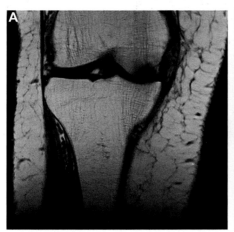
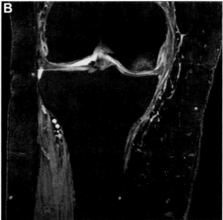

Fig. 13. Coronal T1-weighted (*A*) and DESS (*B*) images demonstrate osteonecrosis of the medial femoral condyle.

commonly with this condition. MR images demonstrate thickening and increased signal intensity at the inferior pole of the patella (Fig. 15). Adjacent marrow edema is not uncommon. Features are appreciated most easily on sagittal images [1,29,31]. Patients who have patellar tendonosis may have associated patellar tracking disorders as well (45%) [33].

Complete tears of the patellar tendon are less common than tendinitis or partial tears. Injury usually occurs with the knee flexed against a contracted quadriceps mechanism. Most tears occur near the patellar attachment [29]. The tendon has a wavy appearance and typically, the patella is retracted to some extent, depending on the degree of knee flexion. Again, sagittal T2-weighted or STIR images are most useful for evaluating this injury (Fig. 16).

Chung and colleagues [35], described the MR features of another patellar tendon condition termed "lateral condyle friction syndrome," which is analogous to the clinical syndrome, fat pad impingement. Patients present with anterior pain with exertion, and focal tenderness over the inferior pole of the patella. MR features include abnormal signal intensity in the soft tissues between the inferior lateral patella and femoral condyle, marrow edema, and abnormal patellar alignment [35].

Patellar retinacular tears

Patellar retinacular injuries are associated most commonly with lateral patellar dislocations [36–39]. The medial soft tissue support of the patella is divided into three layers. The most superficial layer, layer 1, lies just deep to the subcutaneous tissues and is composed of the fascia of the sartorius muscle. Layer 2 lies just deep to layer 1, where the superficial medial ligament fuses anteriorly with

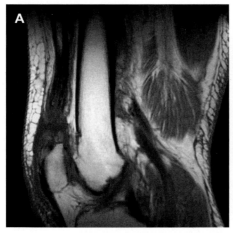
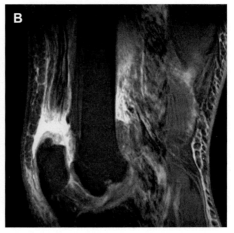

Fig. 14. Third-degree quadriceps strain (complete tear). Sagittal T1- (*A*) and fat-suppressed fast spin-echo T2-weighted (*B*) images demonstrate thickening and high signal intensity through the quadriceps at the patellar attachment.

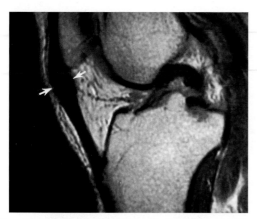

Fig. 15. Patellar tendonosis. Sagittal T1-weighted image demonstrates marked thickening (*arrows*) of the tendon at the patellar attachment.

layer 1 to form the patellar retinaculum, which inserts on the medial margin of the patella [37,38]. Layer 3 forms the joint capsule. Superiorly in layer 2, the medial patellofemoral ligament arises from the medial condyle or adductor tubercle and takes an oblique course deep to the vastus medialis obliquus to insert on the superior two thirds of the medial patellar margin. On axial MR images, the patellar retinaculum is identified as a low signal intensity structure extending from the medial patellar margin and blending with the vastus medialis obliquus fascia [37–39].

Patellar retinaculum tears are almost always medial (94%) and are part of a spectrum of findings associated with lateral patellar dislocations [36]. MR features include joint effusion (55%–100%),

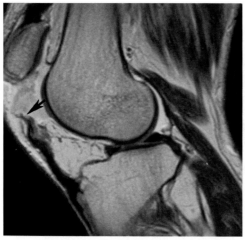

Fig. 16. Complete patellar tendon tear. Sagittal T1-weighted image shows a wavy tendon with complete separation (*arrow*) at the patellar attachment and superior displacement of the patella.

contusions of the anterior lateral femoral condyle (31%–100%), medial patellar facet contusions or osteochondral fractures (41%–61%), patellar tilt (43%), and retinacular complex injuries in 41% to 96% of lateral patellar dislocations (Fig. 17). Tears of the medial patellofemoral ligament occur in up to 96% of patients. Most tears are partial, but up to 40% are complete. Abnormal signal intensity in the vastus medialis obliquus is seen in 45% of cases [38]. Associated injuries include anterior cruciate ligament tears in 18%, and medial collateral ligament and meniscal tears in 11% [36,38]. It is important to detect retinacular complex tears because this indicates surgical repair to avoid the redislocation that occurs in 44% of patients who do not have surgical repair of the retinaculum [37].

Gastrocnemius, soleus, and plantaris injuries

These muscle groups are discussed together because patients are referred commonly to rule out tears of the gastrocnemius when they actually have plantaris muscle tears or associated injuries of the soleus muscle [1,26,40]. The gastrocnemius lies superficially in the calf, with two heads (medial and lateral) arising from the posterior surface of the medial and lateral femoral condyles. The muscle passes distally to join the soleus tendon, forming the Achilles tendon that inserts on the calcaneus [1,26]. Medial gastrocnemius injuries may occur in the mid- or proximal calf, and can be associated with soleus or plantaris strains (Fig. 18). Tears of the lateral gastrocnemius may be associated with popliteus, biceps femoris, and plantaris injury [26].

The plantaris muscle arises from the lateral femur, just above the lateral head of the gastrocnemius. This small muscle has a long tendon that passes distally between the soleus and lateral gastrocnemius to insert on the calcaneus, just anterior to the Achilles tendon [1,26,40]. This muscle is absent in 7% to 10% of patients [40]. Forceful contraction of the plantaris may result in rupture at the myotendinous junction, with possible associated injury to the gastrocnemius, anterior cruciate ligament, and popliteus muscle [26,40].

MR features vary depending on the extent of muscle involvement. Most commonly, there is feathery increased signal intensity in the involved muscle, a common finding in the gastrocnemius. Hematoma formation or fluid collection between the gastrocnemius and soleus also may be evident. The latter is especially common with plantaris tears because the muscle is small and the tendon may not be demonstrated clearly (Fig. 19) [1,40].

Popliteus muscle injuries

The popliteus muscle arises from the posterior medial tibial metaphysis and extends obliquely to

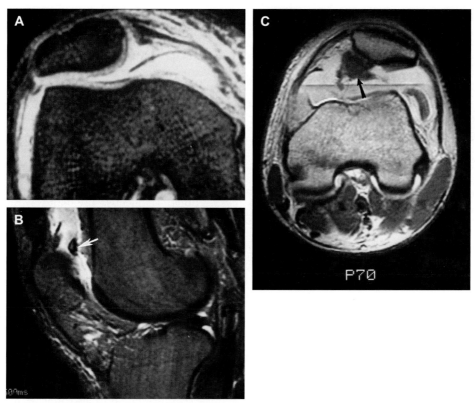

Fig. 17. Lateral patellar dislocations with associated injuries. (*A*) Axial fat-suppressed fast spin-echo T2-weighted image with patellar subluxation and separation at the medial retinacular attachment. (*B*) Sagittal T2-weighted image with an osteochondral fracture (*arrow*) from the superior patella. (*C*) Large effusion with fluid-fluid level and retinacular tear with soft tissue and cartilage debris (*arrow*) in the joint.

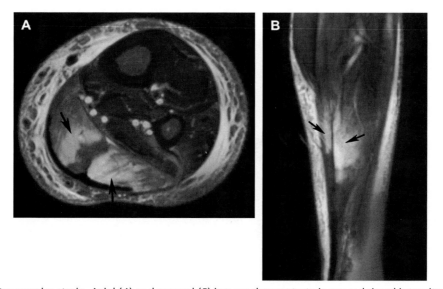

Fig. 18. Gastrocnemius strain. Axial (*A*) and coronal (*B*) images demonstrate increased signal intensity (*arrows*) in the medial and lateral gastrocnemius caused by a first-second degree strain.

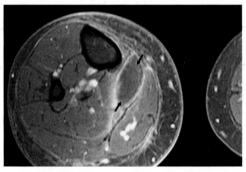

Fig. 19. Plantaris tear. Axial postcontrast fat-suppressed T1-weighed image demonstrates a peripherally enhancing hematoma (*arrows*) between the soleus and gastrocnemius.

insert on the lateral femoral condyle and fibular head. The tendon passes between the capsule and posterior horn of the lateral meniscus [1,26,41]. Once, tears of the popliteus were considered uncommon, but now they are detected more frequently [41]. Tears may involve the body of the muscle or the myotendinous junction. Associated injuries include the posterior cruciate ligament (29%), the anterior cruciate ligament (17%), and bone bruises (33%) [37]. MR features are appreciated most easily on axial and sagittal images, and resemble the injuries described earlier (Fig. 20) [1,41].

Iliotibial band syndrome

The iliotibial band or tract is formed proximally by the fascia of the gluteus maximus and medius and tensor fascia lata. Distally, the iliotibial band attaches to the supracondylar tubercle of the lateral femoral condyle and extends below the joint to insert on Gerdy's tubercle of the tibia [1,26,42,43]. Iliotibial band syndrome, or friction syndrome, is seen in long-distance runners, cyclists, and football players. This syndrome is a common cause of lateral knee pain that may be confused with lateral meniscal tears, lateral collateral ligament injuries, or injuries to the biceps femoris insertion or popliteus muscle [43–46].

MR images demonstrate increased signal intensity deep to the iliotibial band or organized fluid collections. Frequently, the band is thickened, with intermediate signal intensity related to chronic microtrauma (Fig. 21) [1,39–42].

Other myotendinous injuries

The other muscles and tendons about the knee are injured less commonly, especially as isolated strains. The medial tendons (sartorius, gracilis, and semitendinosus) are associated closely because they insert on the anterior tibia forming the pes anserinus. In this group, the sartorius is most prone to injury [26]. In the author's experience, pes anserine bursitis is more common than tendon strain [1].

The semimembranosus also attaches medially at the infraglenoid tubercle of the posterior medial tibia. This tendon may be injured in association with medial gastrocnemius tears. Laterally, the biceps femoris inserts on the head and styloid of the fibula. The biceps femoris is injured commonly in patients who have arcuate ligament tears [47]. MR features are similar to those of other tendon strains. Commonly, biceps femoris strain or

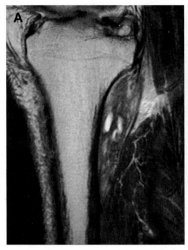
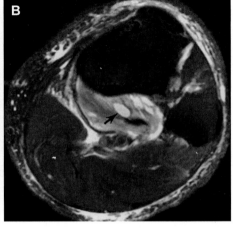

Fig. 20. Popliteus muscle tear. Sagittal T1- (*A*) and axial fat-suppressed fast spin-echo T2-weighted (*B*) images demonstrate diffuse abnormal signal intensity in the popliteus muscle, with a small central hematoma (*arrow in B*).

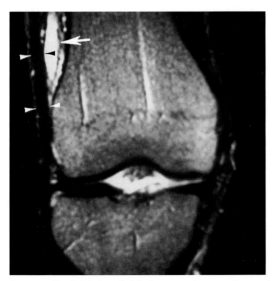

Fig. 21. Iliotibial band friction syndrome. Coronal T2-weighted image shows a fluid collection between the iliotibial band and the femur (*arrow*). Also, the iliotibial band is thickened markedly (*arrowheads*).

avulsion is associated with bone contusion involving the anterior medial femoral condyle [48].

References

[1] Kelley EA, Berquist TH. The knee. In: Berquist TH, editor. MRI of the musculoskeletal system. 5th edition. Philadelphia: Lippincott-Williams and Wilkins; 2006. p. 303–429.

[2] Capps GW, Hayes CW. Easily missed injuries around the knee. Radiographics 1994;14:1191–210.

[3] Futami T, Foster BK, Morris LL, et al. Magnetic resonance imaging of growth plate injuries: the efficacy and indications for surgical procedures. Arch Orthop Trauma Surg 2000;120:390–6.

[4] Sanders TG, Medynski MA, Feller JF, et al. Bone contusion patterns of the knee at MR imaging: footprint for mechanism of injury. Radiographics 2000;20:S135–51.

[5] Williamson RV, Staheli LT. Partial epiphyseal growth arrest: treatment with bridge resection and fat interposition. J Pediatr Orthop 1990;10:769–76.

[6] Eckland K, Jaramillo D. Patterns of premature physeal arrest: MR imaging of 111 children. AJR Am J Roentgenol 2002;178:967–72.

[7] Arndt WF III, Truax AL, Barnett FM, et al. MR diagnosis of bone contusions of the knee: comparison of coronal T2-weighted fast spin-echo with fat saturation and fast spin-echo STIR images with conventional STIR images. AJR Am J Roentgenol 1996;166:119–24.

[8] Palmer WE, Levine SM, Dupuy DE. Knee and shoulder fractures: association of fracture detection and marrow edema on MR images with mechanism of injury. Radiology 1997;204:395–401.

[9] Moosikasuwan JB, Miller TT, Math K, et al. Shifting bone marrow edema of the knee. Skeletal Radiol 2004;33:380–5.

[10] Gaeta M, Minatoli F, Scribano E, et al. CT and MR imaging findings in athletes with early tibial stress injuries: comparison with bone scintigraphic findings and emphasis on cortical abnormalities. Radiology 2005;235:553–61.

[11] Yao L, Johnson C, Gentili A, et al. Stress injuries of bone: analysis of MR imaging staging criteria. Acad Radiol 1998;5:34–40.

[12] Fredericson M, Bergman AG, Hoffman EL, et al. Tibial stress reaction in runners: correlation of clinical symptoms and scintigraphy with a new magnetic imaging grading system. Am J Sports Med 1995;23:472–81.

[13] Holt MK, Williams LA, Dent CM. MRI management of tibial plateau fractures. Injury 1995; 26(9):595–9.

[14] Delzell PB, Schils JP, Recht MP. Subtle fractures about the knee: innocuous-appearing and yet indicative of significant internal derangement. AJR Am J Roentgenol 1996;167:699–703.

[15] Escobedo EM, Mills WJ, Hunter JC. The "reverse Segond" fracture: association with a tear of the posterior cruciate ligament and medial meniscus. AJR Am J Roentgenol 2002;178:979–83.

[16] Huang G-S, Yu JS, Munshi M, et al. Avulsion fracture of the head of the fibula (the "arcuate" sign): MR imaging findings predictive of injuries to the posterolateral ligaments and the posterior cruciate ligament. AJR Am J Roentgenol 2003;180: 381–7.

[17] Beaty JH, Kumar A. Fractures about the knee in children. J Bone Joint Surg Am 1994;76: 1870–80.

[18] Toye LR, Cummings PD, Armendariz G. Adult tibial intercondylar eminence fracture: evaluation with MR imaging. Skeletal Radiol 2002;31: 46–8.

[19] Meyers MH, McKeever FM. Fracture of the intercondylar eminence of the tibia. J Bone Joint Surg Am 1970;52:1677–84.

[20] Bohndorf K. Imaging of acute injuries of the articular surfaces (chondral, osteochondral and subchondral fractures). Skeletal Radiol 1999; 28:545–60.

[21] DeSmet AA, Ilai OA, Graf BK. Reassessment of MR criteria for stability of osteochondritis dissecans in the knee and ankle. Skeletal Radiol 1996; 25:159–63.

[22] Boutin RD, Januario JA, Newberg AH, et al. MR imaging features of osteochondritis dissecans of the femoral sulcus. AJR Am J Roentgenol 2003; 180:641–5.

[23] Norman A, Baker ND. Spontaneous osteonecrosis of the knee and medial meniscal tears. Radiology 1978;129:653–6.

[24] Yamamoto T, Bullough PG. Spontaneous osteonecrosis of the knee: the result of subchondral insufficiency fracture. J Bone Joint Surg Am 2000;82:858–72.

[25] Carpintero P, Leon F, Zafra M, et al. Spontaneous collapse of the tibial plateau: radiological staging. Skeletal Radiol 2005;34:399–404.

[26] Bencardino JT, Rosenberg ZS, Brown RR, et al. Traumatic musculotendinous injuries of the knee: diagnosis with MR imaging. Radiographics 2000;20:S103–20.

[27] May DA, Disler DG, Jones EA, et al. Abnormal signal intensity in skeletal muscle at MR imaging: patterns, pearls and pitfalls. Radiographics 2000;20:S295–315.

[28] Bush CH. The magnetic resonance imaging of musculoskeletal hemorrhage. Skeletal Radiol 2000;29:1–9.

[29] Sonin AH, Fitzgerald SW, Bresler ME, et al. MR imaging appearance of the extensor mechanism of the knee: functional anatomy and injury patterns. Radiographics 1995;15:367–82.

[30] Nance EP, Kaye JJ. Injuries of the quadriceps mechanism. Radiology 1982;142:301–7.

[31] Khan KM, Bonar F, Desmond PM, et al. Patellar tendinosis (Jumper's knee): findings at histopathologic examination, US, and MR imaging. Radiology 1996;200:821–7.

[32] McLoughlin RF, Raber EL, Vellet AD, et al. Patellar tendonitis: MR imaging features, with suggested pathogenesis and proposed classification. Radiology 1995;197:843–8.

[33] Allen GM, Tauro PG, Ostlere SJ. Proximal patellar tendinosis and abnormalities of patellar tracking. Skeletal Radiol 1999;28:220–3.

[34] Ferretti A, Conteduca F, Camerucci E, et al. Patellar tendinosis: a follow-up study to surgical treatment. J Bone Joint Surg Am 2002;84:2179–85.

[35] Chung CB, Skaf A, Roger B, et al. Patellar tendon-lateral femoral condyle friction syndrome: MR imaging in 42 patients. Skeletal Radiol 2001;30:694–7.

[36] Quinn SF, Brown TR, Demlow TA. MR imaging of patellar retinacular ligament injuries. J Magn Reson Imaging 1993;3:843–7.

[37] Spritzer CE, Courneya DL, Burk DL, et al. Medial retinacular complex injury in acute patellar dislocation: MR findings and surgical implications. AJR Am J Roentgenol 1997;168:117–22.

[38] Elias DA, White LM, Fithian DC. Acute lateral patellar dislocation at MR imaging: injury patterns of the medial patellar soft-tissue restraints and osteochondral injuries of the inferomedial patella. Radiology 2002;225:736–43.

[39] Burks RT, Desio SM, Bachus KN, et al. Biomechanical evaluation of lateral patellar dislocations. Am J Knee Surg 1998;11:24–31.

[40] Helms CA, Fritz RC, Garvin GJ. Plantaris muscle injury: evaluation with MR imaging. Radiology 1995;195:201–3.

[41] Brown TR, Quinn SF, Wensel JP, et al. Diagnosis of popliteus injury with MR imaging. Skeletal Radiol 1995;24:511–4.

[42] Nemeth WC, Sanders BL. The lateral synovial recess of the knee: anatomy and role in chronic iliotibial band friction syndrome. Arthroscopy 1996;12(5):574–80.

[43] Muhle C, Ahn JM, Yeh L-R, et al. Iliotibial band friction syndrome: MR imaging findings in 16 patients and MR arthrographic study of six cadaver knees. Radiology 1999;212:103–10.

[44] Nishimura G, Yamoto M, Tamai K, et al. MR findings in iliotibial band syndrome. Skeletal Radiol 1997;26:533–7.

[45] Ekman EF, Pope T, Martin DF, et al. Magnetic resonance imaging of iliotibial band syndrome. Am J Sports Med 1994;22:851–4.

[46] Orchard JW, Fricker PA, Abud AT, et al. Biomechanics of iliotibial band friction syndrome in runners. Am J Sports Med 1996;24:375–9.

[47] Terry GC, La Prade R. The biceps femoris complex at the knee: its anatomy and injury patterns associated with acute anterolateral-anteromedial rotary instability. Am J Sports Med 1996;24:2–8.

[48] Ross G, Chapman AW, Newberg AR, et al. Magnetic resonance imaging for evaluation of acute posterolateral complex injuries of the knee. Am J Sports Med 1997;25:444–8.

RADIOLOGIC
CLINICS
OF NORTH AMERICA

Radiol Clin N Am 45 (2007) 969–982

ELSEVIER
SAUNDERS

MR Imaging of Cysts, Ganglia, and Bursae About the Knee

Francesca D. Beaman, MD[a], Jeffrey J. Peterson, MD[b],*

Cystic lesions around the knee comprise a diverse group of entities, ranging from benign cysts to complications of underlying diseases such as infection, arthritis, and malignancy. Although the presentation of cystic masses may be similar, their management may differ, thus highlighting the importance of appropriate categorization. For the purpose of this article, the authors limit the scope of their discussion to benign cysts, ganglia, and bursae about the knee.

Benign cystic lesions about the knee are common entities encountered in patients of all age groups. Although often discovered as incidental findings, they may present with pain, mechanical dysfunction of the knee, limitation in range of motion, or a palpable mass. Clinical manifestations reflect the size, location, mass effect, and relationship to surrounding structures of a lesion.

MR imaging is recognized as the gold standard in characterizing cystic lesions about the knee because of its ability to image the soft tissues exquisitely. MR can confirm the cystic nature of the lesion, evaluate anatomic relationships, and identify associated intra-articular pathology. In this article, the authors present their experience with benign cystic masses observed about the knee. It is not intended as a comprehensive review, but as an overview, emphasizing those lesions that are more common and highlighting their presentation, histology, pathogenesis, and characteristic MR imaging features.

Synovial cyst

The definition of a synovial cyst is a juxta-articular fluid collection that is lined by synovial cells. It is this synovial lining that histologically distinguishes them from other juxta-articular fluid collections. A synovial cyst represents a focal extension of joint fluid that may, or may not, communicate with the joint, and may extend in any direction [1,2]. The prototypical example of a synovial cyst is the popliteal cyst.

This article was originally published in *Magnetic Resonance Imaging Clinics of North America* 15:1, February 2007.

[a] Center Radiology, PC, Washington Hospital Center, 110 Irving Street NW, Washington, DC 20010, USA
[b] Department of Radiology, Mayo Clinic Jacksonville, 4500 San Pablo Boulevard, Jacksonville, FL 32207, USA
* Corresponding author.
E-mail address: peterson.jeffrey@mayo.edu (J.J. Peterson).

doi:10.1016/j.rcl.2007.08.005

Popliteal (Baker) cyst

A popliteal, or Baker, cyst is the most commonly encountered cyst located about the knee. It is located in the posteromedial aspect of the knee, and represents joint fluid extending through a slit-like communication between the knee joint and the normally occurring gastrocnemius-semimembranosus bursa (Fig. 1) [3,4]. Adult cadaveric studies have shown this communication to be present in more than 50% of the study population [4,5]. In 1877, Baker [6] described eight cases of popliteal fossa swelling and concluded that this finding was secondary to fluid escaping from the knee joint; thus, the term Baker cyst is reserved specifically for a fluid collection in this anatomic location.

In 1972, Wolfe and Colloff [7] outlined two requirements for popliteal cyst formation: an anatomic communication between the knee joint and the gastrocnemius-semimembranosus bursa, and a knee joint effusion. Theories regarding the formation of a popliteal cyst center on the weakness of the posterior joint capsule. The posterolateral joint obtains reinforcement from the ligament of Wisberg, the popliteus tendon, and the posterior cruciate ligament (PCL). Conversely, the posteromedial joint has supplemental reinforcement only from the posterior horn of the medial meniscus attached to the capsule [8]. This relative weakness, in combination with mechanical internal derangement or arthropathy, causes an increase in intra-articular pressure

and a joint effusion, thus allowing joint fluid to escape through the path of lesser resistance into the gastrocnemius-semimembranosus bursa.

The gastrocnemius-semimembranosus bursa is composed of two parts: the gastrocnemius bursa and the semimembranosus bursa. These parts may be separated partially or completely by a central septum. Depending on their intercommunication and the quantity of fluid, one or both of these structures may distend. The semimembranosus bursa is the larger of the two and is located medial to the gastrocnemius component [9]. Classically, a popliteal cyst extends in the inferomedial direction, respecting the intermuscular planes [10]. Although this is the most common appearance, cysts may extend laterally or proximally [2,11], and rarely dissect intramuscularly into the vastus medialis or medial gastrocnemius muscles [10]. A fluid collection deep to the medial gastrocnemius muscle may coincide, representing fluid in the subgastrocnemius bursa [12].

In the literature, the incidence of popliteal cysts in patients who obtain an MR of the knee ranges from 5% to 38% [12–15]. The prevalence increases with age, and is significantly higher in those over 50 years [8]. Statistical association with popliteal cysts has been shown with internal derangement (81%), joint effusion (77%), and degenerative arthropathy (69%) [12]. Tears of the posterior horn of the medial meniscal consistently represent the highest associated derangement, at over 60% [5,7,13]. Fielding and colleagues [13] also showed popliteal cysts coexisting with lateral meniscal tears in 38%, bilateral meniscal tears in 27%, and complete anterior cruciate ligament (ACL) tears in 13% of cases. The posterior horn of the medial meniscus tear is thought to weaken the posterior joint capsule further and provoke an opening into the bursa [13]. Additional associations include prior meniscectomy, collateral or cruciate injury, articular cartilage damage, intra-articular osteochondral loose bodies, osteochondritis dissecans, infection, juvenile rheumatoid arthritis, rheumatoid arthritis, and other arthritides [7,13,16,17]. The presence of an effusion-producing derangement, rather than the abnormality itself, is proposed as the important factor in popliteal cyst formation [7,12]. Similar associations with popliteal cysts have not been shown in the pediatric population. In a review of 393 knee MR examinations in children aged 1 to 17 years, a popliteal cyst was present in 25 (6%), with only 4 of the 25 (16%) having joint effusions, and none with coexisting meniscal or ACL tears [16].

Popliteal cysts can be seen in asymptomatic patients and those presenting with internal or mechanical derangement, pain, a palpable mass,

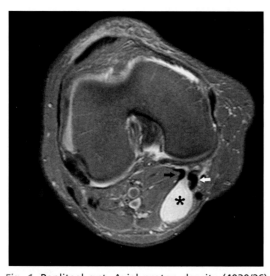

Fig. 1. Popliteal cyst. Axial proton density (4030/26) fast spin echo fat-saturated MR image shows a hyperintense fluid collection (*) in the posteromedial knee, located between the medial gastrocnemius tendon (*black arrow*) and the semimembranosus tendon (*white arrow*).

swelling, or signs and symptoms of thrombophlebitis [7,8,10]. Cysts may rupture and dissect along or into adjacent structures, thus simulating symptoms of thrombophlebitis [8]. Conversely, proximal dissection has been reported to cause compression of the sciatic nerve [18]. Rarely, a deep vein thrombosis may coexist with a dissecting popliteal cyst [8,19]. Calf claudication is also a rare presenting symptom when the popliteal cyst is large and causes extrinsic compression of the popliteal artery [20]. Clinically, popliteal cysts may mimic adipose tissue proliferation, popliteal artery tortuosity or aneurysm, vessel thrombosis, or tumor.

Other synovial cysts

The popliteal cyst is the most common synovial cyst, but it simply represents one specific type of synovial cyst. Synovial cysts about the knee may extend in the anterior, medial, or lateral planes as well [21–23]. The tibiofibular joint communicates with the knee joint in approximately 10% of adults [17]. Although synovial cysts in this location are uncommon, with a reported prevalence of between 0.09% and 0.76% [22,24], they may be associated with pain and foot drop secondary to impingement on the common peroneal nerve [22]. Dysesthesia in the territory of the tibial nerve can also be seen secondary to extension of the synovial cyst into the popliteal fossa [25]. Synovial cysts have also been described deep to the iliotibial band, thus mimicking iliotibial band friction syndrome [21], and deep to the medial patellar retinaculum, causing recurrent medial knee pain postoperatively, following medial meniscus repair [23].

Giant synovial cysts are large, well-defined cavities filled with synovial fluid and lined by a synovium-like membrane, which typically involve large joints such as the knee, shoulder and elbow [26]. Most commonly, these cysts are reported in association with rheumatoid arthritis, but also with trauma, osteoarthritis (OA), gout, systemic lupus erythematosus, and juvenile rheumatoid arthritis [26,27]. Clinical presentation is one of pain and swelling [27].

Imaging features of synovial cysts

A popliteal (Baker) cyst is located in a specific anatomic location, between the tendons of the medial gastrocnemius and semimembranosus muscles, and may extend medial, lateral, superficial, or deep to these muscles [1]. Cysts may be simple, multiloculated, or septated, and contain debris, hemorrhage, or osseous loose bodies (Fig. 2) [1,10,12,17,28]. MR imaging of a simple cyst shows a cystic mass with low signal on T1-weighted and high signal on T2-weighted spin echo or STIR (short-TI inversion-recovery) sequences [1,10,29,30]. Rupture of a cyst typically results in edema in the surrounding fascial planes and subcutaneous fat, with fluid tracking inferiorly along the medial side of the medial gastrocnemius muscle plane (Fig. 3) [17,28]. Blood products from intracystic hemorrhage [28], or protein-rich synovial fluid, may result in increased signal on T1-weighted images. Enhancement may be seen in the cyst wall and internal septations following intravenous gadolinium administration (Fig. 4) [17,28]. Because the cysts are lined by synovium, synovial processes such as synovial osteochondromatosis or pigmented villonodular synovitis may be seen also [12,17], but this is not common. Complex cysts may appear heterogeneous and demonstrate foci

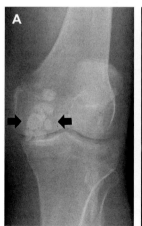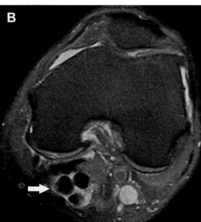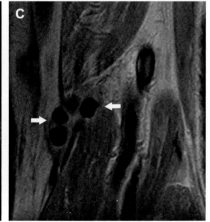

Fig. 2. Loose bodies within a popliteal cyst. (*A*) Anteroposterior radiograph of the knee shows several mineralized loose bodies (*between arrows*) in the medial knee joint. (*B*) Axial T2-weighted (4000/18) fast spin echo fat-saturated and (*C*) coronal T2-weighted fast spin echo MR images show several hypointense loose bodies (*arrows*) within a popliteal cyst.

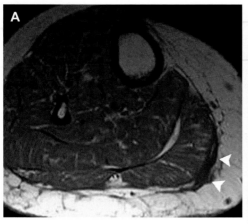

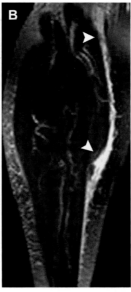

Fig. 3. Popliteal cyst dissection. (A) Axial T1-weighted (819/10) spin echo MR image shows hypointense fluid (*arrowheads*) along the medial margin of the medial gastrocnemius muscle. (B) Coronal T2-weighted (4000/68) fast spin echo fat-saturated MR image nicely shows the extent of the dissected fluid (*arrowheads*) originating from the gastrocnemius-semimembranosus bursa and extending caudally almost the entire length of the calf.

of enhancement following gadolinium administration, thus mimicking neoplasm. Thus, strict adherence to the gastrocnemius – semimembranosus bursal location with communication with the knee joint is essential for accurate diagnosis of a popliteal cyst. An enhancing, solid component suggests a superimposed synovial process.

Ganglion

A ganglion is a cystic, tumor-like lesion of unknown origin, which is surrounded by dense connective tissue filled with gelatinous fluid rich in hyaluronic acid and other mucopolysaccharides [31]. These cysts are classified as myxoid lesions, with suggested causes including synovial herniation and tissue degeneration or repeated trauma [32–34]. The World Health Organization does not address ganglia because they are not tumors, and, therefore, no rigid classification scheme exists. The authors find it useful to place ganglia into one of the following general categories: juxta-articular, intra-articular, and periosteal.

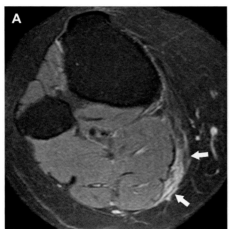

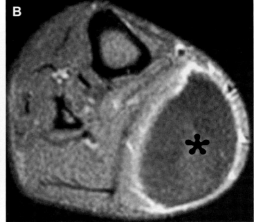

Fig. 4. Popliteal cyst wall enhancement and dissection. (A) Axial proton density (3280/18) fast spin echo fat-saturated MR image shows hyperintense fluid (*arrows*) along the medial gastrocnemius muscle plane, which has dissected caudally from a popliteal cyst. Note the septations within the fluid. (B) Axial T1-weighted (450/11) spin echo fat-saturated, postgadolinium MR image shows a large hypointense cyst (*) juxtaposed between the medial gastrocnemius muscle and subcutaneous tissues. The cyst shows thin rim enhancement following contrast administration.

Juxta-articular ganglion

As a whole, juxta-articular ganglia are quite common, with greater than one half located around the wrist [28]. Around the knee, ganglia may be located in any of the extra-articular soft tissues, and are associated commonly with the origins of the medial and lateral gastrocnemius muscles and the tibiofibular articulation (Fig. 5) [35,36]. Knee lesions are often asymptomatic, discovered incidentally on MR imaging. However, patients may present with pain or symptoms of nerve entrapment, specifically with a lesion arising from the tibiofibular articulation. As with synovial cysts, lesions in this location may compress the common peroneal nerve, resulting in foot drop and paresthesia over the dorsum of the foot [33,37]. If nerve compression is longstanding, MR images may also reveal findings of compressive neuropathy, such as muscle atrophy, fat infiltration, and increased signal on fluid-sensitive sequences.

Intra-articular ganglion

Intra-articular ganglia are relatively uncommon lesions typically associated with the cruciate ligaments, but have also been described in Hoffa's fat pad and arising from the posterior joint capsule [38,39]. The incidence rate on MR imaging is approximately 1% [38,40], which correlates well with the incidence rate reported at arthroscopy of 0.8% to 1.1% [41,42]. Ganglia may be located within or adjacent to the cruciate ligaments [40]. The ACL is affected more commonly than the PCL, with most originating from the tibial insertion of the ACL [38,41]. Although the exact cause of intra-articular ganglia is unknown, they are presumed to be caused by mucinous degeneration of connective tissue. Mucoid degeneration of the cruciate ligament and ganglia likely represent different manifestations along the same pathologic continuum [40]. Another possible theory suggests an origin from herniation of synovial tissue through a defect in the joint capsule or tendon sheath, a mechanism similar to that suggested for wrist ganglia [43].

Intraosseous ganglia are solitary, uni- or multilocular cystic lesions located in the epiphyses of long bones [44]. The pathogenesis is unclear and debate persists as to whether they are distinct from degenerative or posttraumatic cysts. Intraosseous abnormalities frequently coexist with cruciate ganglia and mucoid degeneration of the cruciate ligaments [40]. On MR they are well-defined cystic lesions that may or may not communicate with the joint or be associated with a soft-tissue component [44].

Clinical symptoms are varied but nonspecific, and include knee pain, locking, clicking or popping sensations, and decreased range of motion [38,40,42]. Many patients are asymptomatic, with lesions discovered incidentally on MR or at arthroscopy [41]. Ganglia anterior to the ACL tend to limit knee extension, whereas those posterior to the PCL often limit knee flexion [41].

Periosteal ganglion

Periosteal ganglia are rare lesions, with few described in the literature. More than 50% of periosteal ganglia occur in men, with most patients in

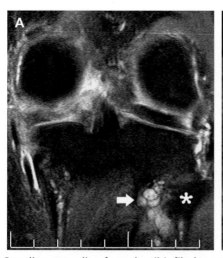
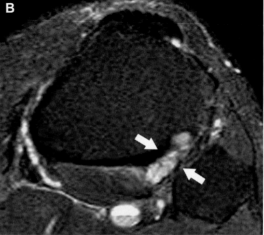

Fig. 5. Ganglion extending from the tibiofibular articulation. (A) Coronal proton density (3527/25) fast spin echo fat-saturated MR image shows a hyperintense, multilobulated fluid collection (*arrow*) extending from the tibiofibular articulation in the soft tissues, just medial to the fibula (*). (B) Axial T2-weighted (2100/68) fast spin echo fat-saturated MR image shows the ganglion to be hyperintense, similar to fluid, and confirms the location in the tibiofibular articulation (*between arrows*).

the fourth or fifth decade. They are found commonly in the region of the pes anserinus, with the remainder located mainly at the ends of long tubular bones [45,46]. As with pes anserine bursitis, patients often present with symptoms mimicking internal derangement of the knee, such as swelling and pain [46].

Imaging features of ganglia

Ganglia may be unilocular or multilocular, are round to lobular in configuration, and often contain sharply defined internal septa. They appear as cystic masses on MR, with low signal intensity on T1-weighted images and high signal intensity on fluid-sensitive and T2-weighted images (Fig. 6) [1,17,29,35,36,38,40]. Long-standing lesions often have a more complex appearance, especially if complicated by previous hemorrhage or infection. Rarely, lesions may be isointense to slightly hyperintense relative to skeletal muscle on T1-weighted images secondary to high proteinaceous content or internal hemorrhage. Following gadolinium administration, rim enhancement may be seen, in addition to diffuse enhancement [40].

Juxta-articular ganglia have features similar to synovial cysts, and thus may be indistinguishable on MR. Making this distinction is of little consequence, with the important features of both entities being location and relationship with adjacent structures. If adjacent to bone, the bone occasionally demonstrates resorption caused by pressure remodeling or periosteal new bone formation (Fig. 7) [34].

Fluid-filled pseudopodia may be seen connecting the ganglia to the adjacent joint.

Anterior cruciate ganglia and mucoid degeneration of the ACL may occur as independent entities or coexist [40], although typically, neither entity is associated with ligamentous instability. Bergin and colleagues [40] proposed criteria for the MR differentiation of ACL ganglia and mucoid degeneration. Criteria for ACL ganglia include fluid signal in the substance of the ligament disproportionate to the quantity of joint fluid, which has a mass effect on intact ligament fibers (Fig. 8). Mucoid degeneration is defined as an intact ligament that is seen poorly on T1-weighted or proton density MR sequences, but seen clearly on T2-weighted sequences [40]. Although ACL ganglia typically have a fusiform appearance and may be interspersed within the fibers of the ligament, posterior cruciate ganglia are typically well-defined cystic structures located along the surface of the ligament (Fig. 9).

Periosteal ganglia typically have a characteristic imaging appearance. The hallmark of these lesions is their associated cortical erosions, caused by extrinsic pressure remodeling [45,46]. Various degrees of cortical scalloping and periosteal new bone formation may also be present, often seen best on radiographs. Spicules of periosteal new bone extend from the scalloped region, oriented perpendicular to the underlying cortex, and appear thick and well-defined [47]. MR shows a juxtacortical mass that is homogeneous and well-defined, with low signal intensity on T1-weighted images and high signal intensity on T2-weighted images [45,46].

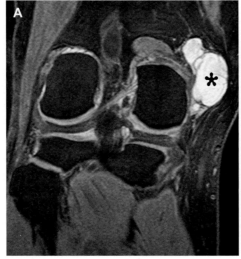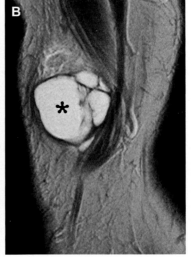

Fig. 6. Ganglion. (*A*) Coronal 3-D double echo steady state (DESS) (22.8/6.22) and (*B*) sagittal T2-weighted (5160/95) fast spin echo MR images show a hyperintense cystic mass (*) in the superomedial knee, compatible with a ganglion. Note the multiple internal septations, which are seen easily on the coronal and sagittal images.

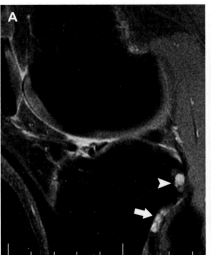
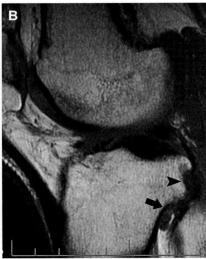

Fig. 7. Juxta-articular ganglion with intraosseous component. (*A*) Sagittal proton density (2650/22) fast spin echo fat-saturated MR image shows a lobulated fluid collection (*arrow*) arising from the tibiofibular articulation and extending along the tibial periosteal margin. Note also the intraosseous component (*arrowhead*) within the posterolateral tibial plateau. (*B*) Sagittal T1-weighted (566.7/11) spin echo MR image shows the periosteal (*arrow*) and intraosseous (*arrowhead*) components of the ganglion to be isointense to skeletal muscle, suggesting proteinaceous or mucinous contents.

Peripheral enhancement may be seen following gadolinium administration [47].

Treatment options for ganglia include excision, puncture, aspiration, and corticosteroid injection. If joint communication exists with juxta-articular or periosteal ganglia, this connection must be excised as well to prevent recurrence.

Subchondral cyst (geode)

Subchondral lucencies are referred to by many names in the literature, including subchondral cysts, synovial cysts, subarticular pseudocysts, necrotic pseudocysts, and geodes [48]. The term subchondral cyst is not accurate technically because the cyst does not have an epithelial lining and is not fluid filled uniformly [48]. However, this term is ubiquitous in the literature, and will therefore be used in the following discussion.

OA is a process of articular degeneration characterized by asymmetric joint space narrowing because of chondromalacia, subchondral bone proliferation, marginal osteophytes, and subchondral lucencies. The pathogenesis of subchondral cyst formation in OA has two prevailing theories. One suggests that elevated intra-articular pressure forces synovial fluid through compromised articular cartilage, with subsequent subchondral cyst formation [49]. The other postulates that the impaction of apposing bony surfaces causes fracture and vascular insufficiency in the subchondral bone, with subsequent cystic necrosis [50]. Degenerative cysts are

often multiple, and segmental in distribution, with surrounding sclerosis and an adjacent abnormal joint. Posttraumatic cysts typically develop over a period of months, have a sclerotic margin,

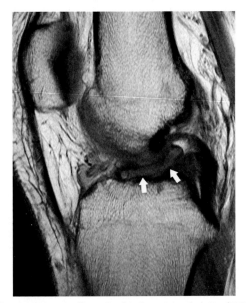

Fig. 8. ACL ganglion. Sagittal proton density (2500/26) fast spin echo MR image shows a fusiform ganglion (*arrows*) with hyperintense signal relative to the PCL, within the intercondylar notch. No intact ACL fibers were present on adjacent images, consistent with a complete ACL tear.

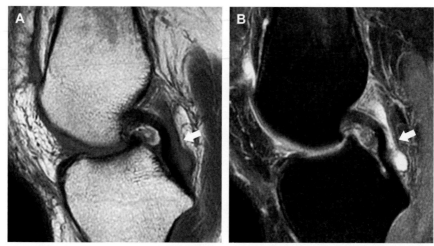

Fig. 9. PCL ganglion. (*A*) Sagittal T1-weighted (616.7/22) SE and (*B*) sagittal proton density (3250/22) fast spin echo MR images show a fusiform fluid collection (*arrow*) posterior to the PCL, which is consistent with a PCL ganglion. T1 signal intensity is isointense to skeletal muscle, suggesting a proteinaceous or mucinous component. Note that there is no associated mucoid degeneration of the PCL.

and communicate with the joint. MR imaging shows focal, nonenhancing fluid collections abutting an articular surface, with a variable degree of associated intra-articular pathology (Figs. 10, 11).

Meniscal cyst

A meniscal cyst is a focal collection of synovial fluid located within, or adjacent to, the meniscus. Various theories have been proposed regarding the etiology of these cysts, with the most widely

accepted reason stating that joint fluid accumulates within a torn or degenerated meniscus, creating an intrameniscal cyst, and fluid extravasation through a meniscal tear into the surrounding soft tissues results in parameniscal cyst formation [30,51,52]. A horizontal component to the tear is present in most cases [17,51]. Although numerous studies have reported lateral meniscal cysts to be two to four times more common than medial meniscal cysts [1,52], additional literature has shown nearly equal cyst frequency between the medial and lateral

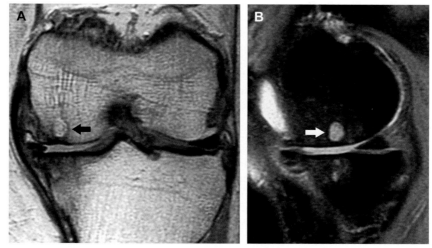

Fig. 10. Subchondral cyst (geode) with OA. (*A*) Coronal proton density (3000/12) fast spin echo and (*B*) sagittal proton density (2366.7/25) fast spin echo fat-saturated MR images show a circumscribed cystic focus (*arrow*) in the distal femur, abutting the articular surface. The 'cyst' is isointense to subcutaneous fat in (*A*), suggesting proteinaceous or mucinous contents. Note the associated osteoarthritic changes of the medial and lateral compartments, with joint space narrowing and osteophytes.

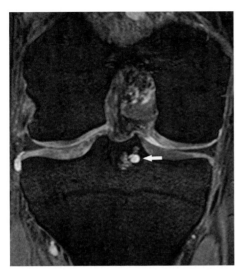

Fig. 11. Subchondral cyst (geode). Coronal 3-D DESS (23.87/6.73) MR image shows a multilobulated hyperintense cyst (*arrow*) in the tibial plateau, abutting the articular surface.

compartments [53], and, also, medial compartment predominance [30,51]. Campbell and colleagues [51] reviewed 2572 imaging reports of knee MR examinations for the prevalence and location of meniscal tears and cysts. They found that medial meniscal tears were twice as common as lateral meniscal tears (66% versus 34%), with a 4% overall prevalence of meniscal cysts (109 cysts in 2572 knees). Two thirds of the cysts were located in the medial compartment, with one third present in the lateral compartment. Although the overall number of medial cysts was greater, the incidence of cysts with respect to the incidence of meniscal tears was equal between the compartments (7.7% medially and 7.8% laterally). Tschirch and colleagues [30] conducted a review of MR images in 102 asymptomatic knees and also observed medial meniscal cyst predominance, with 4 cases having medial cysts and no cases with lateral cysts.

Most meniscal cysts are associated with tears of the associated meniscus, with up to 98% of cases demonstrating a direct communication identifiable on MR imaging (Fig. 12) [51]. In those cases where no distinct connection can be identified, one may see a meniscal tear with no communication to the cyst, or a degenerative intrasubstance signal within the meniscus, which does not meet strict MR imaging criteria for a tear [30,51]. The location of meniscal cysts is determined by the location of the meniscal tear and the capsuloligamentous planes of the knee [17,54]. Most medial cysts are located posteromedially [54], adjacent to the posterior horn [51], but may also be primarily located anteriorly, adjacent to the anterior horn, next to the meniscal body, or may extend superficial to the medial collateral ligament (MCL) [51,54]. Lateral cysts are more varied, with one study showing 54% adjacent to the anterior horn, 16% adjacent to the body, and 30% adjacent to the posterior horn [51]. Anteriorly, the cysts may track deep to

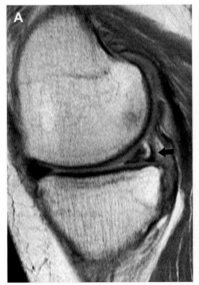
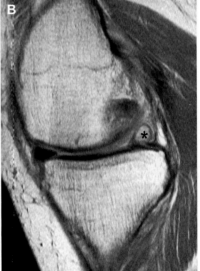

Fig. 12. Meniscal cyst. Consecutive sagittal proton density (3000/25) fast spin echo MR images show a tear in the posterior horn of the medial meniscus (*arrow in A*) and a cyst (* *in B*) extending into the intercondylar notch through this defect. Note the cyst is hyperintense to skeletal muscle, suggesting proteinaceous or mucinous contents.

the iliotibial band, and posteriorly, they may track deep to the lateral collateral ligament [54]. Pericruciate meniscal cysts, which arise from the posterior horn of the medial meniscus tears, simulate PCL ganglia because of their location posterior to, or surrounding, this structure. Differentiation may be important clinically, owing to differences in treatment options. Four MR findings of pericruciate meniscal cysts that may aid in the differentiation include (1) identification of a meniscal tear, (2) connection between the torn meniscus and the cyst, (3) location mainly posterior to the PCL and centered on the ligament, or (4) location surrounding the PCL. PCL ganglia tend to be located at the femoral or tibial insertion of the PCL, rarely surround the ligament, and do not communicate with a meniscal tear, should one be present [55].

Patients typically present with symptoms including swelling, a palpable mass, pain and tenderness, or limited mobility [1,29,55], although asymptomatic cysts may be detected as well [30]. Lateral meniscal cysts present as palpable masses more commonly than medial meniscal cysts [17,51], likely because of the relatively scant amount of fatty soft tissue present in the lateral aspect of the knee [51]. On MR imaging, a well-circumscribed cystic mass is seen, which may be unilocular or show septations and multiple loculations with low signal intensity on T1-weighted images, and increased signal intensity on T2-weighted images [1,17,29,51,55,56]. Cyst contents may also be isointense to skeletal muscle on T1-weighted images secondary to hemorrhage or high proteinaceous content, or low signal on T2-weighted images because of hemosiderin deposition or content desiccation [17,52,56]. Meniscal cysts may also result in osseous erosions [57,58]. Therapy typically requires both cyst drainage and repair of the associated meniscal tear.

Bursa

Bursae are normally occurring, synovial-lined structures that function to reduce friction between moving structures, such as tendons, ligaments, and bone. Typically, they are not visible on imaging because they normally contain only limited fluid. Inflammation from local and systemic processes such as overuse, trauma, internal joint derangement, inflammatory arthropathy, and collagen vascular diseases, in addition to infection and hemorrhage, may cause thickening of the synovial lining and fluid accumulation [1,17]. In this scenario, the bursae become visible on MR imaging as fluid collections with low signal on T1-weighted images and high signal on T2-weighted images. In chronic cases, signal may be more heterogeneous, and complicated by hemorrhage and calcification, thus mimicking a soft-tissue tumor [2,59]. Acute inflammatory bursitis usually responds to rest, ice, and nonsteroidal anti-inflammatory medications, whereas chronic bursitis may require aspiration, local anesthetic, or corticosteroid injections. Infectious bursitis necessitates aspiration and antibiotic therapy [1,17].

Bursae about the knee are numerous and normally occurring. Discussing them based on anatomic location (anterior, posterior, medial, or lateral) provides a useful means of classification. Anterior and posterior bursae are demonstrated best on sagittal or axial images, whereas medial or lateral bursae are seen best on coronal or axial images.

Anterior

The suprapatellar bursa is a midline structure that is located between the quadriceps tendon and the femur. It normally communicates with joint, unless the suprapatellar plica, a normal embryonic septum, fails to involute, thus isolating this compartment (Fig. 13) [1]. Clinically, patients may

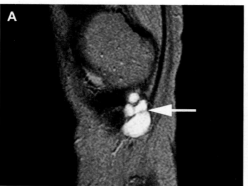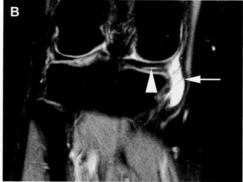

Fig. 13. Meniscal cyst. (*A*) Sagittal T2 (4050/79) fast spin echo and (*B*) coronal fat-suppressed proton density (3000/25) MR images depict a horizontal tear (*arrowhead*) of the medial meniscus with an associated complex medial meniscal cyst (*arrows*).

present with an anterior soft-tissue mass caused by bursal enlargement because of fluid accumulation from synovitis, hemorrhage, or trauma [1]. Loose bodies arising from the joint may be isolated within this compartment, especially if the septum is discontinuous.

The prepatellar bursa is located anteriorly between the patella and subcutaneous tissues. Bursitis is caused commonly by overuse injury or chronic trauma, such as occupational or recreational kneeling or crawling (housemaid's knee, carpet-layer's knee), and results in focal pain and swelling. On MR, a focal fluid collection is seen anterior to the patella. It may be heterogeneous or poorly defined on T2-weighted images, from associated inflammation, hemorrhage, or even infection [1].

The superficial infrapatellar, or pretibial, bursa is juxtaposed between the tibial tubercle and the overlying skin. Although this is an uncommon site of bursitis, direct trauma or occupational overuse (clergyman's knee) may result in focal inflammation or hemorrhage, causing pain anterior to the tibial tubercle [1,17].

The deep infrapatellar bursa is located directly posterior to the distal third of the patellar tendon, juxtaposed between the tendon and the anterior tibia. Cadaveric study has shown no connection with the knee joint, and an average width slightly greater than the width of the distal patellar tendon [60]. Normally, a small amount of fluid may be seen in this bursa on MR imaging [30,61]. Conversely, deep infrapatellar bursitis results from extensor mechanism overuse, particularly in runners and jumpers, and manifests as anterior knee pain, mimicking patellar tendonitis [60].

Posterior

The gastrocnemius-semimembranosus bursa, or popliteal cyst, is discussed in the synovial cyst section.

Medial

The pes anserine bursa is located along the medial aspect of the tibia and separates the pes anserinus, which is formed by the distal tendons of the sartorius, gracilis, and semitendinosus muscles, and the distal tibial collateral ligament at the tibial insertion [1,9,17]. The prevalence of pes anserine bursitis on MR has been shown at 2.5% in symptomatic cases, whereas the prevalence of fluid in the bursa, without clinical symptoms of bursitis, has been shown to be as high as 5%, thus allowing investigators to conclude that not all fluid-containing bursae represent bursitis [30,62]. Pes anserine bursitis frequently results from overuse injury, often in runners, causing medial knee pain and swelling. Pes anserine bursitis commonly mimics a medial

meniscus tear clinically [62]. On MR, a fluid collection is identified along the medial joint, adjacent to the pes anserinus, which does not communicate with the joint. Meniscal and synovial cysts may also occur in a similar location, but they do communicate with the joint, although this communication is not always visible [1].

The MCL, or tibial collateral ligament, bursa is a vertically elongated compartment located between the superficial and deep layers of the MCL, at the level of the middle knee joint line (Fig. 14). Cadaveric study has shown separate femoral and tibial components in most specimens [63]. Fluid confined to the MCL bursa as an isolated finding is extremely rare, with most cases associated with arthridities (OA, gout, rheumatoid) and medial intra-articular pathology [17,63]. Additionally, edema surrounding the MCL has been associated with OA and medial intra-articular pathology [64].

The semimembranosus-tibial collateral ligament bursa, also located along the medial joint line, lies between the semimembranosus tendon and the MCL, at the level of the medial tibial condyle. Inflammation may result in focal pain along the posteromedial knee at the level of the knee joint line. The MR appearance is that of a fluid collection oriented along the plane of the semimembranosus tendon, which may drape over or surround the tendon [29]. This bursa does not communicate with

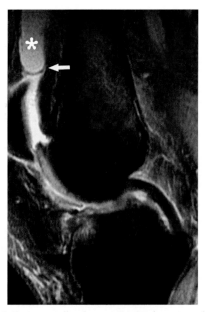

Fig. 14. Suprapatellar bursa. Sagittal proton density (3000/26) fast spin echo fat-saturated MR image shows a suprapatellar bursa (*), which normally communicates with joint unless the suprapatellar plica (*arrow*) fails to involute, thus isolating this compartment.

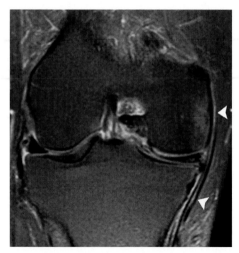

Fig. 15. MCL bursa. Coronal proton density (2610/44) fast spin echo fat-saturated MR image shows hyperintense signal (*arrowheads*) between the superficial and deep layers of the MCL, consistent with MCL bursal fluid. Note this patient had experienced recent medial knee trauma, with resultant medial meniscus tear and medial femoral condyle bone contusion.

the knee joint or other medial knee bursa, although multifocal bursitis may coexist. The proximal extent of the bursa abuts the posterior horn of the medial meniscus; thus, a meniscal cyst is in the differential for a fluid collection in this location [65].

Lateral

The iliotibial band bursa is located between the distal portion of the iliotibial band, just proximal to its insertion on Gerdy's tubercle, and the adjacent tibia. Overuse injury, commonly in runners, is the leading cause of bursal inflammation, with resultant anterolateral knee pain. MR shows a well-defined fluid collection near the insertion of the iliotibial band on the tibia. Clinically, bursitis may mimic iliotibial tendonitis, with the latter condition showing abnormal MR signal within the tendon itself [1].

The fibular collateral ligament (FCL)-biceps femoris bursa is located lateral to the distal FCL, and extends around the anterior and anteromedial portions of this ligament. Cadaveric study has shown a consistent anatomic location, with the superior extent at the level of the crossing of the biceps femoris superficial to the FCL, and the distal extent at the insertion of the FCL on the fibular head [66].

Summary

Cystic lesions about the knee are common findings, representing diverse causes and, therefore, varied prognosis and therapeutic options. MR aids in the

characterization of lesions by first localizing them, and then defining their relationship with adjacent structures and identifying any additional abnormalities. Cystic lesions and their relationships are best depicted on long TE/TR (fluid-sensitive) MR sequences. Careful attention to these details will allow one to provide a reasonable MR diagnosis and thus ensure the most appropriate patient care.

References

[1] Janzen DL, Peterfy CG, Forbes JR, et al. Cystic lesions around the knee joint: MR imaging findings. AJR Am J Roentgenol 1994;163:155–61.

[2] Steiner E, Steinbach LS, Schnarkowski P, et al. Ganglia and cysts around joints. Radiol Clin North Am 1996;34:395–425.

[3] Lindgren PG, Willen R. Gastrocnemio-semimembranosus bursa and its relation to the knee joint. Anatomy and histology. Acta Radiol 1977;18:497–512.

[4] Lindgren PG, Willen R. Gastrocnemio-semimembranosus bursa and its relation to the knee joint. II. Post mortem radiography. Acta Radiol 1977;18:698–704.

[5] Wilson PD, Eyre-Brook AL, Francis JD. A clinical and anatomic study of the semimembranosus bursa in relation to popliteal cyst. J Bone Joint Surg Am 1938;20:963–84.

[6] Baker WM. On the formation of synovial cysts in the leg in connection with disease of the knee-joint. 1877. Clin Orthop Relat Res 1994;299:2–10.

[7] Wolfe RD, Colloff B. Popliteal cysts. An arthrographic study and review of the literature. J Bone Joint Surg Am 1972;54:1057–63.

[8] Labropoulos N, Shifrin DA, Paxinos O. New insights into the development of popliteal cysts. Br J Surg 2004;91:1313–8.

[9] Lee KR, Cox GG, Neff JR, et al. Cystic masses of the knee: arthrographic and CT evaluation. AJR Am J Roentgenol 1987;148:329–34.

[10] Fang CSJ, McCarthy CL, McNally EG. Intramuscular dissection of Baker's cysts: report on three cases. Skeletal Radiol 2004;33:367–71.

[11] Torreggiani WC, Al-Ismail K, Munk PL, et al. The imaging spectrum of Baker's (popliteal) cysts. Clin Radiol 2002;57:681–91.

[12] Miller TT, Staron RB, Koenigsberg T, et al. MR imaging of Baker cysts: association with internal derangement, effusion and degenerative arthropathy. Radiology 1996;201:247–50.

[13] Fielding JR, Franklin PD, Kustan J. Popliteal cysts: a reassessment using magnetic resonance imaging. Skeletal Radiol 1991;20:433–5.

[14] Marti-Bonmati L, Molla E, Dosda R, et al. MR imaging of Baker cysts – prevalence and relation to internal derangement of the knee. MAGMA 2000;10:205–10.

[15] Stone KR, Stoller D, De Carli A, et al. The frequency of Baker's cysts associated with meniscal tears. Am J Sports Med 1996;24(5):670–1.

[16] De Maeseneer M, Debaere C, Desprechins B, et al. Popliteal cysts in children: prevalence, appearance and associated findings at MR imaging. Pediatr Radiol 1999;29:605–9.

[17] McCarthy CL, McNally EG. The MRI appearance of cystic lesions around the knee. Skeletal Radiol 2004;33:187–209.

[18] Robertson CM, Robertson RF, Strazerri JC. Proximal dissection of a popliteal cyst with sciatic nerve compression. Orthopedics 2003;26: 1231–2.

[19] Lazarus ML, Ray CE, Maniquis CG. MRI findings on concurrent acute DVT and dissecting popliteal cyst. Magn Reson Imaging 1994;12: 15–158.

[20] Zhang WW, Lukan JK, Dryjski ML. Nonoperative management of lower extremity claudication caused by a Baker's cyst: case report and review of the literature. Vascular 2003;4:244–7.

[21] Costa ML, Marshall T, Donell ST, et al. Knee synovial cyst presenting as iliotibial band friction syndrome. Knee 2004;11:247–8.

[22] Hersekli MA, Akpinar S, Demirors H, et al. Synovial cysts of the proximal tibiofibular joint causing peroneal nerve palsy: report of three cases and review of the literature. Arch Orthop Trauma Surg 2004;124:711–4.

[23] Nakamae A, Masataka D, Yasumoto M, et al. Synovial cyst formation resulting from nonabsorbable meniscal repair devices for meniscal repair. Arthroscopy 2004;20:16–9.

[24] Ilahi OA, Younas SA, Labbe MR, et al. Prevalence of ganglion cysts originating from proximal tibiofibular joint: a magnetic resonance imaging study. Arthroscopy 2003;19:150–3.

[25] Sansone V, Sosio C, da Gama Malcher M, et al. Two cases of tibial nerve compression caused by uncommon popliteal cysts. Arthroscopy 2002;18:1–3.

[26] Fedullo LM, Bonakdarpour A, Moyer RA, et al. Giant synovial cysts. Skeletal Radiol 1984;12: 901–96.

[27] Rubman MH, Schultz E, Sallis JG. Proximal dissection of a popliteal giant synovial cyst: a case report. Am J Orthop 1997;26:33–6.

[28] Krandorf MJ, Murphey MD (Eds). Synovial tumors. In: Imaging of soft tissue tumors. 2nd edition. Lippincott Williams and Wilkins, Philadelphia. 2006. p. 381–436.

[29] Beall DP, Ly JQ, Wolff JD, et al. Cystic masses of the knee: magnetic resonance imaging features. Curr Probl Diagn Radiol 2005;34: 143–59.

[30] Tschirch FTC, Schmid MR, Pfirrmann CWA, et al. Prevalence and size of meniscal cysts, ganglionic cysts, synovial cysts of the popliteal space, fluid-filled bursae, and other fluid collections in asymptomatic knees on MR imaging. AJR Am J Roentgenol 2003;180:1431–6.

[31] Tom BM, Rao VM, Farole A. Bilateral temporomandibular joint ganglion cysts: CT and MR characteristics. AJNR Am J Neuroradiol 1990;11: 746–8.

[32] Conrad EU, Enneking WF. Common soft tissue tumors. Clin Symp 1990;42:21.

[33] Kili S, Perkins RDP. Common peroneal nerve ganglion following trauma. Injury 2004;35: 938–9.

[34] Weiss SW, Goldblum JR. Benign tumors and tumor-like lesions of synovial tissue. In: Strauss M, editor. Enzinger and Weiss's soft tissue tumors. 4th edition. St. Louis (MO): Mosby; 2001. p. 1037–62.

[35] James SL, Connell DA, Bell J, et al. Ganglion cysts at the gastrocnemius origin: a series of ten cases. Skeletal Radiol 2007;36:139–43.

[36] Bianchi S, Abdelwahab IF, Kenan S, et al. Intramuscular ganglia arising from the superior tibiofibular joint: CT and MR evaluation. Skeletal Radiol 1995;24:253–6.

[37] Iverson DJ. MRI detection of cysts of the knee causing common peroneal neuropathy. Neurology 2005;65:1829–31.

[38] Bui-Mansfield LT, Youngberg RA. Intraarticular ganglia of the knee: prevalence, presentation, etiology, and management. AJR Am J Roentgenol 1997;168:123–7.

[39] Tachibana Y, Ninomiya T, Goto T, et al. Intraarticular ganglia arising from the posterior joint capsule of the knee. Arthroscopy 2004; 20:54–9.

[40] Bergin D, Morrison WB, Carrino JA, et al. Anterior cruciate ligament ganglia and mucoid degeneration: coexistence and clinical correlation. AJR Am J Roentgenol 2004;182:1283–7.

[41] Krudwig WK, Schulte KK, Heinemann C. Intraarticular ganglion cysts of the knee joint: a report of 85 cases and review of the literature. Knee Surg Sports Traumatol Arthrosc 2004;12:123–9.

[42] Parish EN, Dixon P, Cross MJ. Ganglion cysts of the anterior cruciate ligament: a series of 15 cases. Arthroscopy 2005;21:445–7.

[43] Angelides AC, Wallace PF. The dorsal ganglion of the wrist: its pathogenesis, gross microscopic anatomy and surgical treatment. J Hand Surg Am 1976;1:228–35.

[44] Bancroft LW, Peterson JJ, Kransdorf MJ. Cysts, geodes and erosions. Radiol Clin North Am 2004;42:73–87.

[45] Okada K, Unoki E, Kubota H, et al. Periosteal ganglion: a report of three new cases including MRI findings and a review of the literature. Skeletal Radiol 1996;25:153–7.

[46] Abdelwahab IF, Kenan S, Hermann G, et al. Periosteal ganglia: CT and MR imaging features. Radiology 1993;188:245–8.

[47] De Maeseneer M, De Boeck H, Shahabpour M, et al. Subperiosteal ganglion cyst of the tibia. A communication with the knee demonstrated by delayed arthrography. J Bone Joint Surg Br 1999;81:643–6.

[48] Resnick D (Ed). Degenerative disease of extraspinal locations. In: Bone and joint disorders. 4th edition, WB Saunders, Philadelphia. 2002. 1271–381.

[49] Freud E. The pathological significance of intra-articular pressure. Edinburgh Med J 1940;47: 192.

[50] Rhaney K, Lamb DW. The cysts of osteoarthritis of the hip: a radiologic and pathologic study. J Bone Joint Surg Br 1955;37:663.

[51] Campbell SE, Sanders TG, Morrison WB. MR imaging of meniscal cysts: incidence, location, and clinical significance. AJR Am J Roentgenol 2001; 177:409–13.

[52] Tyson LL, Daughters TC Jr, Ryu RKN, et al. MRI appearance of meniscal cysts. Skeletal Radiol 1995;24:421–4.

[53] Tasker AD, Ostlere SJ. Relative incidence and morphology of lateral and medial meniscal cysts detected by magnetic resonance imaging. Clin Radiol 1995;50:778–81.

[54] De Maeseneer M, Shahabpour M, vanderdood K, et al. MR imaging of meniscal cysts: evaluation of location and extension using a three-layer approach. Eur J Radiol 2001;39:117–24.

[55] Lektrakul N, Skaf A, Yeh L, et al. Pericruciate meniscal cysts arising from tears of the posterior horn of the medial meniscus: MR imaging features that simulate posterior cruciate ganglion cysts. AJR Am J Roentgenol 1999;172: 1575–9.

[56] Berquist TH (Ed). Knee. In: MRI of the musculoskeletal system. 5th edition. Lippincott Williams and Wilkins, Philadelphia. 2006. p. 303–429.

[57] Blair TR, Schweitzer M, Resnick D. Meniscal cysts causing bone erosion: retrospective analysis of seven cases. Clin Imaging 1999;23:134–8.

[58] Juhng SK, Lenchik L, Won JJ. Tibial plateau erosions associated with lateral meniscal cysts. Skeletal Radiol 1998;27:288–90.

[59] Stahnke M, Mangham DC, Davies AM. Calcific hemorrhagic bursitis anterior to the knee mimicking a soft tissue sarcoma: report of two cases. Skeletal Radiol 2004;33:363–6.

[60] LaPrade RF. The anatomy of the deep infrapatellar bursa of the knee. Am J Sports Med 1998;26: 129–32.

[61] Aydingoz U, Oguz B, Aydingoz O, et al. The deep infrapatellar bursa. J Comput Assist Tomogr 2004;28:557–61.

[62] Rennie WJ, Saifuddin A. Pes anserine bursitis: incidence in symptomatic knees and clinical presentation. Skeletal Radiol 2005;34:395–8.

[63] De Maeseneer M, Shahabpour M, Van Roy F, et al. MR imaging of the medial collateral ligament bursa: findings in patients and anatomic data derived from cadavers. AJR Am J Roentgenol 2001;177:911–7.

[64] Blankenbaker DG, De Smet AA, Fine JP. Is intra-articular pathology associated with MCL edema on MR imaging of the non-traumatic knee? Skeletal Radiol 2005;34:462–7.

[65] Rothstein CP, Laorr A, Helmes CA, et al. Semimembranosus-tibial collateral ligament bursa: MR imaging. AJR Am J Roentgenol 1996;166: 875–7.

[66] LaPrade RF, Hamilton CD. The fibular collateral ligament-biceps femoris bursa. An anatomic study. Am J Sports Med 1997;25:439–43.

RADIOLOGIC CLINICS OF NORTH AMERICA

Radiol Clin N Am 45 (2007) 983–1002

Magnetic Resonance Imaging of the Collateral Ligaments and the Anatomic Quadrants of the Knee

Douglas P. Beall, MD[a],*, J. David Googe, MD[b],
Jason T. Moss[c], Justin Q. Ly, MD[d], Barry J. Greer, MD[d],
Annette M. Stapp, RN, BSN[e], Hal D. Martin, DO[f]

The supporting structures providing stability to the medial and lateral portions of the knee have been an area of interest long before the advent of MR imaging and the initial dissections were performed to gain additional anatomic understanding of these regions to perform successful surgical repairs [1,2]. An optimal surgical repair of medial and/or lateral supporting structures is necessary, because deficient ligaments in these regions can contribute to rotational instability of the knee [3–5].

Evaluation with MR imaging of the medial and lateral structures of the knee is effective but remains challenging because of the anatomic variation and the thin nature of most of these structures [6,7]. The difficult nature of the anatomy emphasizes the need to be familiar with the normal anatomic appearance of the structures located in these regions. The normal anatomy represents a complex of supporting structures working together to provide dynamic and static stability. The goal of

This article was originally published in *Magnetic Resonance Imaging Clinics of North America* 15:1, February 2007.

[a] Clinical Radiology of Oklahoma, 610 NW 14th Street, Oklahoma City, OK 73103, USA

[b] Department of Orthopedics, University of Oklahoma Health Science Center, 1012 NW 41st, Oklahoma City, OK 73118, USA

[c] Texas Tech University College of Medicine, NW 6114 10th Drive, Lubbock, TX 79416, USA

[d] Department of Radiology, Wilford Hall Medical Center, 2200 Bergquist Drive, Suite 1, Lackland AFB, TX 78236-5300, USA

[e] Clinical Radiology of Oklahoma, 1828 NW 177th Terrace, Edmond, OK 73003, USA

[f] Oklahoma Sports Science & Orthopaedics, 6205 N. Santa Fe, Suite 200, Oklahoma City, OK 73118, USA

* Corresponding author.

E-mail address: dpb@okss.com (D.P. Beall).

doi:10.1016/j.rcl.2007.08.006

postinjury or preoperative assessment with MR imaging is to identify the primary anatomic elements that are injured along with any secondary supporting structures that may be damaged [6,7].

The collateral ligaments are defined elements and are often depicted in anatomic texts as isolated bands extending from the femur to the tibia; but it has been known for nearly three decades that there is significant anatomic complexity in these regions. This complexity has more recently lead to considering injuries to these regions as posterolateral corner or posteromedial corner injuries in addition to injuries to the ligaments themselves [1–3,8]. Optimal modern surgical planning is based upon physical examination in combination with accurate MR imaging anatomic evaluation to detect the associated injuries found in these regions and address them appropriately [8,9]. An anatomic assessment based on MR imaging alone will provide some information, but combing the knowledge of normal anatomy, injury patterns, and how best to display the medial and lateral collateral ligaments (LCLs) provides the greatest amount of information and assistance to the treating physician.

The description of the injury and its location is also important. Though many of these injuries are complex and may involve many associate structures, the knee may be divided into quadrants including the posterolateral corner, the anterolateral knee, the posteromedial corner, and the anteromedial knee. The quadrants refer to the periphery of the knee joint as opposed to the central portion of the knee joint, which is primarily occupied by the cruciate ligaments. It is common to have associated injuries of the cruciate ligaments, but this division helps with description organization and accurate communication of injury information. This manuscript discusses the anatomy of the four quadrants, provides cadaveric and imaging examples of these quadrants, describes the most common mechanisms of injury, and gives various examples of injuries to the various anatomic structures located within these quadrants of the knee.

Anatomy

Lateral collateral ligament/posterolateral corner

The anatomy of the posterolateral corner of the knee is complex and contains many important ligaments, tendons muscles, and their associated osseous structures. The stabilizing structures include the LCL, the popliteus muscle and tendon, the arcuate ligament, the popliteofibular ligament, the popliteomeniscal fascicles, the oblique popliteal ligament, the tendons of the short and long heads of the biceps femoris, the fabellofibular ligament,

and the lateral gastrocnemious muscle. Most of the structures of the posterolateral corner are best seen in the coronal plane (ie, the LCL, the arcuate ligament, the popliteofibular ligament, the fabellofibular ligament, and the tendons of the short and long heads of the biceps femoris) or the axial plane (ie, the popliteus muscle and tendon, and oblique popliteal ligament) but some of the anatomy is best demonstrated on the sagittal plane (ie, the popliteomeniscal fascicles and the lateral gastrocnemious muscle) (Figs. 1–3). A coronal oblique scanning orientation has also been described for improved visualization of the popliteofibular ligament, the arcuate ligament, and the fabellofibular ligament (Fig. 4) [10].

The LCL itself comprises components from the capsule, the biceps femoris, and the iliotibial band [11,12]. Nearly all tears of the LCL are associated with damage to posterolateral corner structures. There are authors that divide the LCL into a fibular collateral ligament located more posteriorly and an LCL proper (a vertically oriented thickening of the lateral capsule at its midpoint) located more anteriorly (Fig. 5) [12]. A structure known as the anterior oblique band (AOB) has also been described as a band of fibrous tissue that originates from the fibular collateral ligament and extends inferiorly and obliquely to attach to the lateral portion of the tibia. The AOB blends with posterior fibers of the iliotibial tract (ITT) (Fig. 6).

There is also some variability in the terminology used to describe the anatomy of the posterolateral corner. Be aware that there may occasionally be a discrepancy in the names of some of the structures in this location. Notably, the popliteofibular ligament has also been referred to as the short external lateral ligament, the popliteofibular fascicle, and the fibular origin of the popliteus muscle [13,14]. Adhering to standard nomenclature will improve communication accuracy when describing anatomic structures, and the use of standard terms should be applied whenever possible.

Anterolateral knee

Anterolateral stabilizers primarily include the knee joint capsule, the ITT, and the AOB of the fibular collateral ligament that joins the fibular collateral ligament to the iliotibial band (see Figs. 5 and 6). An early description of the connection between the posterolateral and anterolateral knee was made by Johnson [15] who reported prominent interdigitating fibers that connected the LCL to the ITT 2 cm above the insertion of the ITT on the lateral tibial plateau. This connection also functions to stabilize the lateral portion of the knee as tension on the ITT is transmitted through both the LCL and to the attachment site of the ITT (Gerdy's tubercle) [15].

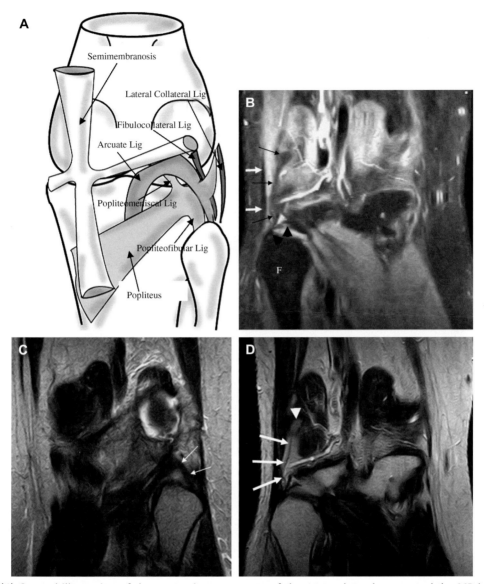

Fig. 1. (*A*) Coronal illustration of the anatomic components of the posterolateral corner and the MR imaging correlates as demonstrated by coronal proton density–weighted MR images with fat saturation (*B*) and coronal T2–weighted MR images without fat saturation (*C, D*). (*B*) Coronal T2–weighted proton density image with fat saturation demonstrates the LCL (fibular collateral ligament portion) (*black arrows*), the arcuate ligament (*black arrowheads*), and the tendons of the short and long heads of the biceps femoris (*white arrows*). F, fibula. (*C*) Coronal T2–weighted image shows the popliteofibular ligament (*white arrows*). (*D*) Coronal T2–weighted MR image shows the fabellofibular ligament (*white arrows*). The fabella is also seen on this image (*white arrowhead*).

The anterolateral knee structures and their relationship to the other lateral components of the knee have been described by other authors who have divided the anatomic components into layers. Seebacher and colleagues [2] described three layers of the lateral portion of the knee and grouped the anterolateral knee structures with the components of the posterolateral corner. The layers were divided into: a superficial layer, layer 1, which comprised the ITT anteriorly and the biceps femoris posteriorly; layer 2, which contained the quadriceps retinaculum anteriorly; and layer 3, which was formed by the lateral joint capsule extending from the patella to the posterior cruciate ligament. The authors described two laminae that originate from the capsule. The superficial lamina was found to contribute to the fibular collateral ligament and the fabellofibular ligament, and the deep lamina

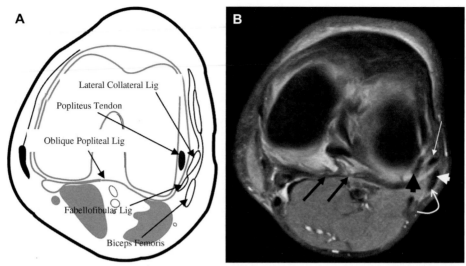

Fig. 2. (*A*) Axial illustration of the anatomic components of the posterolateral corner and the MR imaging correlate as demonstrated by an axial proton density–weighted MR image with fat saturation. (*B*) Axial illustration of the anatomic components of the posterolateral corner and the MR imaging correlates as demonstrated by axial T2–weighted MR images with fat saturation and shows the oblique popliteal ligament (*black arrows*) and the popliteus tendon (*black arrowhead*) as well as the LCL (*white arrow*). The components of the biceps femoris can also be demonstrated at this level including the direct arm of the short head of the biceps tendon (*curved white arrow*), which is posterior and slightly medial to the direct and anterior arms of the long head of the biceps tendon (*white arrowhead*).

was found to form the coronary ligament (also known as the meniscofemoral and meniscotibial ligaments) and the popliteal hiatus, as well as the arcuate ligament. Terry and colleagues [16] described five layers: aponeurotic, superficial, middle, deep, and capsulo-osseous layers with interdigitation between the various layers.

In addition to the AOB attachment to the lateral tibia, there is also a broad insertion of fibers originating from the ITT that attach to the lateral tibia posterior to Gerdy's tubercle (Fig. 7). The attachment of the ITT, the AOB, and other fibers originating from these structures is well seen in MR imaging (Fig. 8).

Medial collateral ligament/posteromedial corner

The medial collateral ligament (MCL) is often depicted as a simple band-like structure in some anatomic texts but rather is a ligamentous structure that is comprised of three layers and blends imperceptibly with the surrounding structure of the posteromedial and anteromedial knee. Knowledge of the normal appearance of these anatomic structures and their relationship to one another may serve to accurately assess the degree of injury present and to predict the presence of associated injuries. The accurate preoperative MR imaging assessment of injury to this region can assist in optimal surgical repair and restoration of optimal function [17].

Medial and posteromedial structures include the medial collateral ligament, the posterior oblique ligament (POL), the semimembranosis tendon, the medial head of the gastrocnemius muscle, and the oblique popliteal ligament. The medial and posteromedial structures are well demonstrated on MR imaging (Fig. 9). When evaluating the medial and posteromedial structures of the knee, the axial and coronal planes are most useful (see Fig. 9, Fig. 10), and a coronal oblique plane has been described as being optimal for the evaluation of the POL (Fig. 11) [6].

Early investigation of the medial portion of the knee involved categorizing the anatomic structures into three layers. Warren and Marshall [1] conducted an anatomic study involving 154 fresh frozen cadaver specimens and defined a crural fascia layer, a superficial medial ligament layer, and a capsular layer. Superficially, the MCL blends in with the crural fibers and connects to the fascia of the medial retinaculum and the vastus medialis anteriorly and is continuous with the posterior capsule and semimembranosis posteriorly while attaching to the medial portion of the medial meniscus. The layer classification has been preserved in a modified version and can be applied to cadaver dissections as well as to MR images (Figs. 12–14).

The POL is a structure that has been well described from cadaveric dissections and extends from the medial tubercle to the posterior portion of the capsule where the superior arm attaches

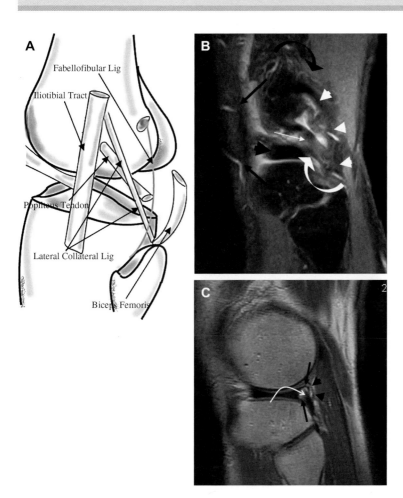

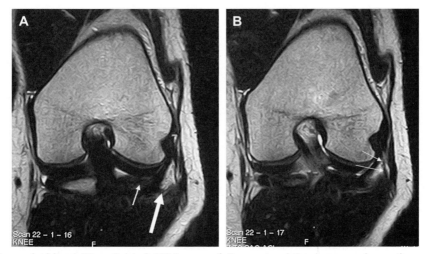

Fig. 3. (A) Sagittal illustration of the anatomic components of the posterolateral corner. (B) The sagittal proton density MR image with fat saturation demonstrates the biceps femoris tendon (white arrowheads) and the LCL (straight white arrow) immediately adjacent to the distal biceps femoris tendon. The iliotibial band (black arrows), the popliteal tendon (curved white arrow), and the lateral meniscus (black arrowhead) are also well visualized. A portion of the lateral head of the gastrocnemius is also apparent on this single sagittal image (curved black arrow). (C) A sagittal proton density–weighted MR image shows the superior and inferior popliteomeniscal ligaments (black arrows) surrounding the popliteus tendon (curved white arrow) as well as the arcuate ligament more posteriorly (black arrowheads).

Fig. 4. (A) Coronal oblique T2–weighted MR image of the posterolateral corner shows the popliteofibular ligament (larger white arrow) and the popliteomeniscal ligament (smaller white arrow). (B) Coronal oblique T2–weighted MR image shows the arcuate ligament (white arrows) as it extends inferiorly to attach to the proximal fibula.

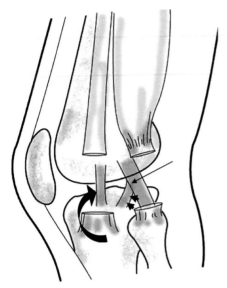

Fig. 5. Sagittal diagram representation demonstrating the separate anatomic components of the LCL and the fibular collateral ligament. The AOB (*black arrowheads*) is seen to extend anteriorly and inferiorly from its proximal attachment on the fibular collateral ligament (*black arrow*). There are authors that divide the LCL into a fibular collateral ligament located more posteriorly (*black arrow*) and an LCL proper (a vertically oriented thickening of the lateral capsule at its midpoint) located more anteriorly (*curved black arrow*).

to the joint capsule and the proximal portion of the oblique ligament and the inferior arm attaches to the semimembranosis tendon sheath (Fig. 15).

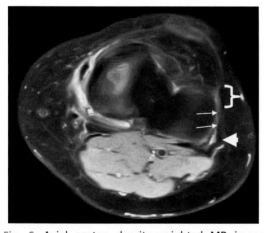

Fig. 6. Axial proton density–weighted MR image demonstrating the fibular collateral ligament (*white arrowhead*), the iliotibial band (*white bracket*), and the AOB of the fibular collateral ligament (*white arrows*) that extends from the fibula to attach to the lateral midtibia and blends with fibers from the posterior portion of the iliotibial band.

Anteromedial knee

The medial and anteromedial knee is comprised of the anterior portion of the MCL, the patellar retinaculum, and the medial patellofemoral ligament (MPFL) (see Fig. 9, Fig. 16). The fibers of layer 2 as described by Warren and Marshall [1] are split vertically just anterior to the MCL. The fibers anterior to this split extend superior to the vastus medialis and merge with layer 1 to form the patellar retinaculum. The fibers posterior to the split contribute to the MCL and contribute to the MPFL that runs from the vastus medialis tubercle deep to the vastus medialis to attach to the superior portion of the patella (Fig. 17).

A normal variation is a medial patellar plica that extends from the medial patellar retinaculum/joint capsule attach to the synovium covering the infrapatellar fat pad (see Fig. 15). The medial patellar plica has been classified into four types (A through D), based on size with the larger types (C and D) more likely to produce symptoms [18].

Mechanism of injury/MR imaging appearance

Posterolateral corner

Posterolateral corner injuries are not as common as injuries to the medial supporting structures of the knee, but patients who have lateral ligamentous

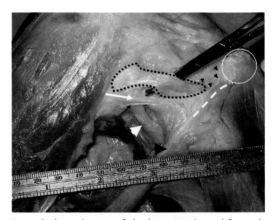

Fig. 7. Cadaver image of the knee as viewed from the lateral side demonstrates the LCL (*border defined by dotted line*) that is lifted up by the hemostat instrument, the distal biceps femoris (*large black arrowhead*), the lateral head of the gastrocnemius (*white arrowhead*), the arcuate ligament (*black arrow*), the fabellofibular ligament (*white arrow*), distal ITT fibers attaching to Gerdy's tubercle (*area within white circle*), and fibers extending anteriorly from the LCL and posteriorly from the ITT (*small black arrowheads*) to attach to the proximal tibial rim (*white dashed line*). The fibers extending anteriorly from the LCL are part of the AOB.

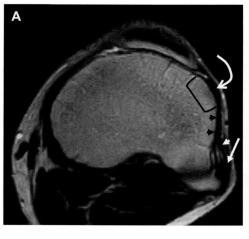

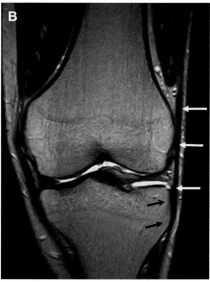

Fig. 8. (*A*) Axial T2–weighted MR image through the proximal tibia shows the attachment of the ITT (*curved white arrow*) to Gerdy's tubercle (*black bracket*). The fibular collateral ligament is also seen as a condensation of fibers just anterior to the fibular head (*white arrow*). Fibers from the ITT (*black arrowheads*) and from the AOB (*white arrowhead*) are also seen to attach to the lateral rim of the proximal tibia. (*B*) Coronal T2–weighted MR image shows the ITT (*white arrows*) along the lateral portion of the knee and its attachment to Gerdy's tubercle (*black arrows*).

damage are more likely to have coexisting injuries to the cruciate ligaments and medial knee structures. Injuries to the posterolateral corner often result from an abrupt external rotation of the tibia in an extended knee, from a posterolaterally directed impact to the medial portion of the proximal tibia or from a hyperextension injury. When a severe posterolateral corner injury is encountered, its detection may be clinically difficult, because the

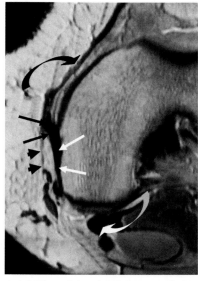

Fig. 9. Axial T2–weighted MR image of the medial knee shows the MCL (*black arrows*), the POL (*white arrows*), the crural fibers (*black arrowheads*), the medial retinaculum (*curved black arrow*), and the semimembranosis tendon (*curved white arrow*).

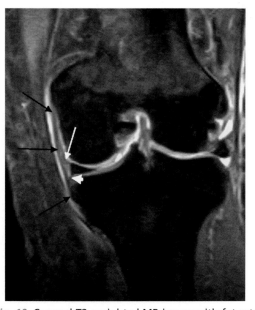

Fig. 10. Coronal T2–weighted MR image with fat saturation shows the superoinferior extent of the MCL (*black arrows*) and the deep layer of the MCL, including the meniscofemoral (*white arrow*) and the meniscotibial ligaments (*white arrowhead*).

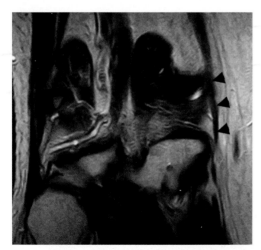

Fig. 11. Coronal oblique T2–weighted MR image shows the posterior oblique ligament (*black arrowheads*). This ligament is seen in its entirety from superior to inferior because of the oblique coronal orientation of the image.

presence of associated cruciate ligament injuries may make an accurate physical examination difficult [19]. Isolated injuries to the posterolateral corner are uncommon and are also difficult to detect on physical examination. Patients typically present with minor trauma (ie, a hyperextension injury) with posterolateral knee pain and a sensation of knee instability in extension. Physical examination often reveals posterolateral knee tenderness and/or ecchymosis. A high index of suspicion is necessary in patients who have posterolateral knee pain because chronic deficiency of these supporting structures can lead to chronic posterolateral rotational instability and/or subsequent failure of cruciate ligament reconstruction [3,20].

Posterolateral corner injuries are complex and may involve several different anatomic structures. Initial postinjury imaging evaluation typically begins with conventional radiographs. The radiographs are most often negative for fracture but can demonstrate a subtle avulsion fracture of the superior portion of the fibular head. This avulsion fracture is usually shaped like an arc of bone and is known as the arcuate sign when seen on the radiograph (see Fig. 16) [21]. This sign has been described as being pathognomonic for injury to the posterolateral corner and has been linked to posterolateral knee instability [22]. An avulsion fracture involving only the styloid process of the fibula has been seen to involve structures located more medially in the posterolateral corner, including the arcuate ligament and the popliteofibular ligament (Fig. 18). Even if direct visualization of injury to these structures is not evident, a styloid process avulsion fracture or bone marrow edema in this location implies injury to these structures [22]. An avulsion fracture of the lateral aspect of the fibular head is associated with injury to the conjoined tendon (including the fibular collateral ligament and the biceps femoris tendon). The fragment, with this fracture, is typically larger and is associated with a greater amount of marrow edema [22].

Almost all tears of the LCL are associated with other injuries. These injuries include damage to structures within the region of the LCL, such as the capsule, the biceps femoris, and the popliteus, as well as to structures elsewhere in the knee, such as the cruciate ligaments or the lateral tibial rim (Segond fracture) (Fig. 19).

The popliteus muscle is the main lateral stabilizer of the knee and is also involved in internal rotation

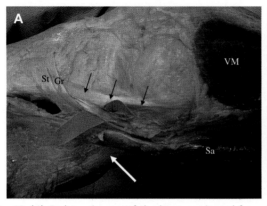
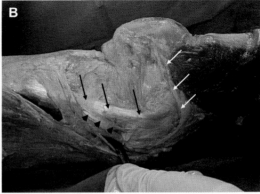

Fig. 12. (*A*) Cadaver image of the knee as viewed from the medial side shows the POL (isolated with blue tape passed under it), the MCL (*black arrows*), the medial head of the gastrocnemius (*white arrow*), the semitendinosus (St), the gracilis (Gr), the sartorius (Sa), and the vastus medialis (VM). (*B*) Cadaver image of the knee as viewed from the medial side shows the POL (*black arrowheads*), the MCL (*black arrows*), and the MPFL (*white arrows*).

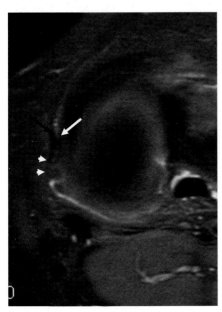

Fig. 13. Axial T2–weighted MR image of the medial knee with fat saturation shows the three layers of the MCL including layer 1 (*white arrowheads*), layer 2 (*black arrow*), and layer 3 (*white arrow*).

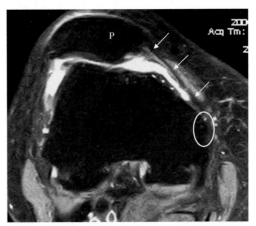

Fig. 15. Axial T2–weighted MR image of the right knee demonstrates the MPFL (*white arrows*) extending from the vastus medialis tubercle (*area within circle*) to medial border of the superior patella (P).

of the knee. Forced lateral rotation and/or varus stress can injure the popliteal tendon that usually tears at or near the musculotendinous junction (Fig. 20). The popliteomeniscal ligament also provides posterolateral stability and prevents anterior subluxation of the meniscus during knee extension. Rupture of these ligaments can cause instability of the lateral meniscus and have been associated with lateral meniscal tears (Fig. 21) [23]. The popliteofibular ligament acts to stabilize the popliteus muscle and tendon. These associated injuries are commonly seen with injury to the popliteus muscle and tendon, as less than 10% of popliteal injuries are isolated [24,25].

The appearance of the posterolateral corner injuries at MR imaging depends upon what structures are injured and the degree of injury. Disruption of the ligaments may occur proximally, distally, or in the mid portion of the ligament. A complete ligamentous disruption appears as a disruption of all of the fibers comprising the ligament (see Fig. 19), whereas a partial disruption is characterized by disruption of a portion of the ligament

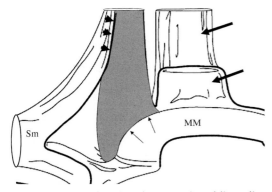

Fig. 14. Diagram showing the posterior oblique ligament (POL) (*dark gray shaded area*) and its attachment to the posteromedial portion of the medial meniscus (*small black arrows*), medial meniscus (MM), the semimembranosis (Sm) (*black arrowheads*), and the MCL (*large black arrows*).

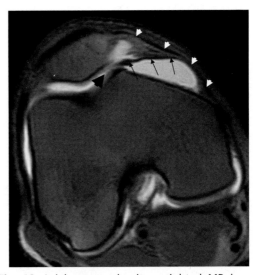

Fig. 16. Axial proton density weighted MR image obtained after the injection of 35 mL of dilute gadolinium shows a medial patellar plica extending from the medial patellar retinaculum (*white arrowheads*) toward the medial patellofemoral joint (*black arrowhead*).

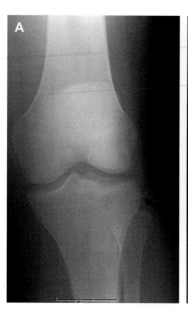
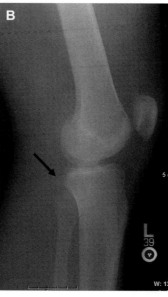

Fig. 17. (*A, B*) Anteroposterior and lateral conventional radiographs of the left knee reveal an avulsion fracture superior to the fibular head (*black arrows*) consistent with an arcuate sign in this patient who was brought into the emergency department by ambulance after a motor vehicle accident.

and areas of fluid signal within the substance of the ligament itself [26]. A minor ligament injury where there is a sprain injury (but without identifiable fiber disruption) has been described as a grade 1 injury [27]. The grading classification is most commonly applied to tears of the MCL, but the spectrum of injury from a mild sprain injury to complete ligamentous disruption may be applied to all ligament injuries.

Similar to ligamentous injury, the MR imaging appearance of tendon injuries depends on the site and degree of injury. Most commonly the tendon will tear at the musculotendinous junction, which is a relative site of weakness for most musculotendinous units (Fig. 20A, B), but a tendon may tear at its site of attachment or distally, just proximal to its attachment site. The posterolateral corner contains the biceps femoris tendon as well as the popliteus tendon, both of which may be injured and torn (see Figs. 19 and 20). Complete tears may also have a component of tendon retraction that is most often seen as a tear of the distal tendon and proximal retraction of the torn tendon and muscle. This retracted soft tissue can be seen as a mass and should not be mistaken for a neoplasm

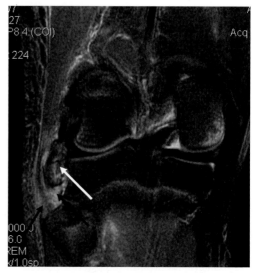

Fig. 18. Sagittal T2–weighted MR image with fat saturation demonstrates a tear of the arcuate ligament (*black arrow*). This patient was also noted to have a tear of the LCL and a small avulsion fracture of the styloid process of the fibula (not shown).

Fig. 19. Coronal T2–weighted MR image with fat saturation demonstrate a complete tear of the LCL (*white arrow*) as well as a near complete tear of the biceps femoris tendon (*black arrows*) at its insertion point.

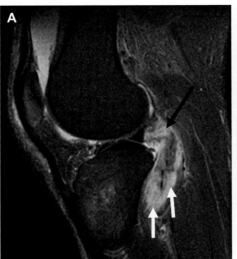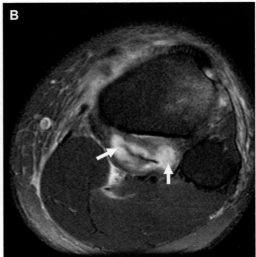

Fig. 20. (A) Sagittal and (B) axial T2-weighted MR images with fat saturation show edema (*white arrows in A and B*) surrounding a musculotendinous junction rupture of the popliteus (*black arrow in A*).

especially when the tendon tear is chronic and the initial injury may have been forgotten or not correctly diagnosed [28]. Any fluid signal (on the fluid-sensitive MR imaging sequences) in or around the tendon should initiate close evaluation of the tendon for detecting a tendon tear.

Anterolateral knee

The structures of the anterolateral quadrant are more frequently injured compared with the components of the posterolateral corner, and anterolateral injuries are usually associated with tears of the anterior cruciate ligament (ACL). The structures of the anterolateral knee are most commonly injured after a varus force (acute stress on the lateral portion of the knee) combined with forceful internal rotation.

The most common location of injury in the anterolateral knee is the posterior fibers of the ITT. These fibers are often interdigitated with, and connected to, the AOB. The AOB extends between the fibular collateral ligament and the ITT and inserts on the lateral portion of the tibia (see Fig. 5). This interconnection and attachment site has also been suspected as being a contributor to the bony avulsion fracture of the lateral tibial rim known as a Segond fracture [29].

This fracture was originally described by a French surgeon, Paul Ferdinon Segond (1851–1912) and is one of the most common injuries of the anterolateral knee. The Segond fracture is thought to result from a traction injury when varus stress and internal rotation forces on the ITT and the AOB cause a tibial avulsion injury (Fig. 22). On MR imaging, the avulsed cortical fragment may not be evident, but marrow edema is commonly noted at the site

of the avulsion. The Segond fracture is also associated with other injuries most of the time (see Fig. 22), and the mechanism of injury that produces this fracture leads to associated ACL tears in 75% to 100% of patients and medial meniscal tears in 66% to 75% [30–32]. Tearing of the lateral knee joint capsule may also occur and chronic

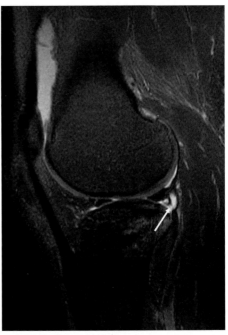

Fig. 21. Sagittal T2–weighted MR image with fat saturation demonstrates a tear of the inferior popliteomeniscal ligament (*white arrow*).

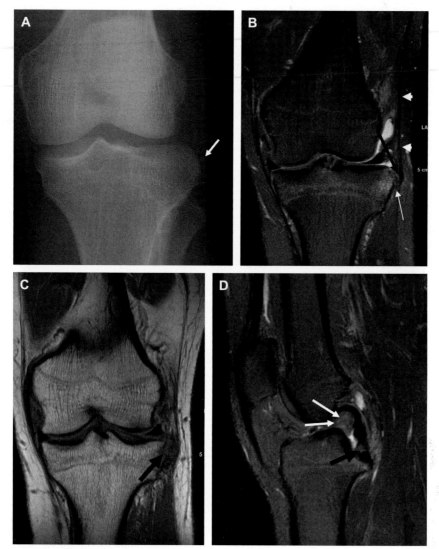

Fig. 22. (*A–D*) The lateral tibial avulsion fracture that is the hallmark of the Segond fracture is demonstrated by conventional radiography (*white arrow in A*). A coronal T2–weighted MR image with fat saturation demonstrates the avulsion fracture (*white arrow in B*), the fibers of the ITT (*white arrowheads*), and their attachment to the fracture fragment (*black arrow*). The coronal T1–weighted image shows the fracture defect where the avulsion fracture fragment has been displaced from the lateral tibial rim (*black arrow in C*). A sagittal T2–weighted MR image with fat saturation (*D*) shows associated injuries, including a complete ACL tear with the absence of any normal ACL fibers (*white arrows in D*) along with a partial tear of the distal posterior cruciate ligament (*black arrow in C*).

anterolateral rotary instability may develop if the injury is untreated.

The Segond injury and other injuries to the ITT, the AOB, and the lateral tibial rim are best seen on the coronal MR images. The fluid-sensitive sequences are best at demonstrating the tears of the distal tendon and ligamentous fibers, and the fracture itself is most optimally seen on the T1-weighted images (see Fig. 22). Other similar injuries such as an avulsion fracture of Gerdy's

tubercle are also well seen on MR imaging but are best seen on the sagittal and axial images (Fig. 23).

Medial collateral ligament/posteromedial corner

MCL is an important stabilizer of the medial portion of the knee. Injuries to this region typically occur from contact, most often a blow to the lateral aspect of the knee or proximal tibia [5]. This contact typically results in an external rotation and

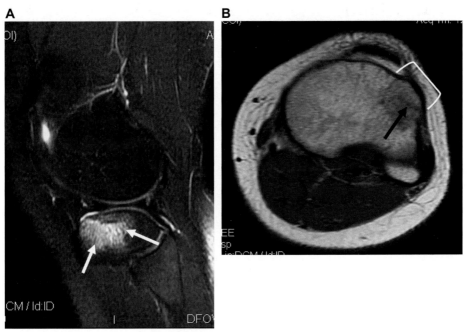

Fig. 23. (*A, B*) Fracture of Gerdy's tubercle. Sagittal (*A*) T2-weighted MR image with fat saturation demonstrates a region of increased signal in the lateral and anterior tibial plateau (*white arrows in A*). Axial T1–weighted MR image (*B*) shows a linear area of decreased signal (*black arrow in B*) extending medially from the lateral and posterior border of Gerdy's tubercle (*white bracket*).

abduction force to the flexed knee with the foot remaining on the ground. Injuries to the medial and posteromedial aspect of the knee may also result from a blow to the anterolateral portion of the tibia, from direct posterior blow to the tibia, and from noncontact twisting injuries [5].

The POL is necessary for optimal stability of the posteromedial knee and has been shown to be functionally independent of the MCL [17]. Injuries to the POL generally occur as a result of forces that are similar to those that injure the MCL. When the knee is unstable in extension, this physical examination finding is consistent with a POL tear. The POL is generally taut in extension and less so in flexion, but the ligament tension is increased somewhat in flexion by the contraction of the semimembranosis [17]. This anatomic configuration allows the POL to contribute to both static and dynamic stability of the medial knee.

Due to the proximity of the POL to the MCL, the medial stabilizing role of the POL and the similarities of mechanism injury to the MCL, the POL is usually involved in injuries to the medial knee that result in tears of the MCL. Injury to the POL is important to recognize because an adequate repair is necessary for appropriate medial knee stability.

The traditional classification of MCL tears is to grade the damage as first- through third-degree sprain/tear injuries. A first-degree tear of the MCL corresponds to ligamentous fibers that are stretched but that are intact (Fig. 24A). First-degree MCL injuries are not associated with increased medial laxity on physical examination. Second-degree MCL tears are characterized by partially intact ligamentous fibers and increased laxity on physical examination (Fig. 24B). The laxity, however, is associated with a definable endpoint. A third-degree MCL tear has complete fiber disruption with medial knee instability and no endpoint on physical examination (Fig. 24C).

There is often overestimation of the presence of an MCL injury given that there may be other pathologic processes that will give rise to fluid surrounding the MCL. Processes including osteoarthritis, chondromalacia, meniscal tears, parameniscal cysts, or MCL bursitis will contribute to fluid surrounding the MCL and can provide confusion as to the presence or absence of an MCL injury in patients who have traumatic medial knee pain. Although the value of the MCL injury grading system can be limited in grading low-grade injuries, it is helpful with third degree MCL tears because the frank ligamentous disruption is usually evident on the coronal and axial MR images.

A careful evaluation of the MR imaging examination must be performed because isolated injuries to MCL are unusual and most injuries involve

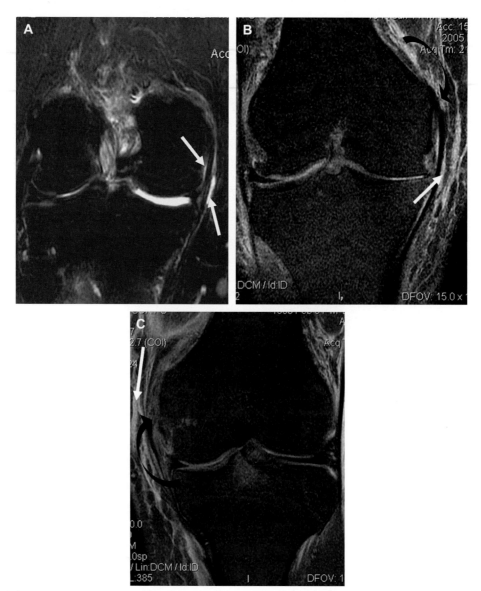

Fig. 24. (*A*) Coronal T2–weighted MR image with fat saturation shows fluid surrounding the medial collateral ligament (MCL) (*white arrows*) but no evidence of ligament fiber disruption. This appearance is consistent with a first-degree MCL injury in this patient who sustained a sharp blow to the lateral portion of the knee. (*B*) Coronal T2–weighted MR image with fat saturation demonstrates a second-degree MCL injury with fluid surrounding the MCL (*white arrow*) and partial disruption of the fibers of the superior portion of the MCL (*black curved arrow*). (*C*) Coronal T2–weighted MR image with fat saturation reveals a third degree MCL injury with complete disruption of the proximal MCL (*black curved arrow*) and fluid surrounding the medial ligamentous structures of the knee (*white arrow*).

other structures surrounding the MCL. The most common injuries associated with MCL tears are ACL tear, medial meniscal tears (O'Donoghue's unhappy triad), meniscocapsular separations, medial retinaculum disruption, POL tears, tears of the semimembranosis, vastus medialis tears, and disruption of the posteromedial knee joint capsule.

The MR imaging evaluation should also include close scrutiny of the medial meniscus, especially in regard to medial extrusion of the medial meniscus. Extrusion is defined as pathologic displacement of the meniscus of more than 3 mm beyond the central margin of the medial tibial plateau [33]. A weight-bearing MR imaging investigation has drawn an association with displaceable meniscal tears and MCL lesions [34]. The authors reported that patients who had displaceable meniscal tears had significantly more pain than patients who had nondisplaceable meniscal tears independent of any other abnormalities. They also found that grade 2 or 3 MCL tears were present in all of the displaceable meniscal tears but only in 12% of the nondisplaceable tears. The medial meniscus is important to evaluate in conjunction with the MCL because higher-grade MCL tears are often associated with medial displacement of the meniscus, and this displacement may be more likely related to patient symptoms (ie, pain).

The location of MCL tears is also important to identify. The MCL is most optimally visualized in its entirety on the coronal sequences and edema (indicative of MCL injury) is best noted on the fluid-sensitive sequences (Fig. 24). The axial plane is also optimal for cross-sectional evaluation of the MCL. In an MCL tear, there is typically increased signal within the ligament itself without an associated knee joint effusion (unless there is another injury such as an associated ACL tear or patellar dislocation).

The location is important to identify because tears in different locations may be treated differently [35,36]. Tears from the femoral origin are the most common type of tear and are often associated with a bony avulsion fragment and may be treated with reattachment to the femur by way of suture anchors or screws. Ligament disruption in the mid portion of the ligament are typically repaired with end-to-end suturing, and tears of the distal portion of the MCL may involve the pes anserine tendons and can be reattached to bone with sutures or stapling.

The MR imaging examination is also important to scrutinize for other associated injuries such as an ACL tear. An ACL tear will cause additional de-stabilization of the joint, and it may be necessary to wait until the MCL tear is healed before performing an ACL reconstruction [35,36]. An exception to this might be if a proximal MCL tear was accompanied by a bony avulsion and could be repaired primarily along with an ACL reconstruction.

The MR imaging appearance of an MCL tear is important to evaluate, because nonoperative healing potential is directly related to the size of the gap between torn ends of the MCL [35,36]. The optimal healing potential of the MCL is well known, and the healing time typically correlates with the degree of MCL injury. The MR evaluation may provide additional clinical evidence on which method may be most likely to successfully treat a particular MCL tear. Thickening or minimal redundancy of the MCL may be present on the post-injury images after the ligament has healed, and these findings typically do not correlate to ligament weakness or medial laxity. The thickened ligament represents scar tissue that is less than the strength of the native MCL, but the load to failure is typically unchanged as the amount of scar tissue is greater than the thickness of the original ligament [37].

The MR imaging evaluation of the POL is similar to that of the MCL but the POL may better evaluated by using a coronal oblique plane. This plane is prescribed from a sagittal MR localizer sequence and is typically a 25-degree posterior oblique plane along the superoinferior course of the POL (Fig. 25).

The POL is also most commonly torn at its proximal portion and may heal well if the torn ends are in reasonably close proximity. The coronal and axial images are the most optimal planes for evaluation of the POL (Fig. 26). An accurate evaluation of the POL is important just as it is for the MCL because it can reveal the severity of the injury, can reveal any associated injuries (ie, tears of the semimembranosis or MCL), and can assist the surgeon in planning a repair if it is necessary. Some authors have suggested that repair of POL tears may improve long-term stability and resistance to static and dynamic valgus stress.

Anteromedial knee

The anterior fibers of the MCL, the ACL, and the medial meniscus are important for maintaining stability of the anteromedial knee. Flexion and torsional forces are important for producing the injuries to these structures. The injury is most often caused by a pivoting and twisting action (common in such sports as skiing, basketball, football, soccer, lacrosse, and tennis). When the body is moving forward with one foot in contact with the ground, external rotation, valgus, and flexing forces are normally applied to the knee [5]. This force is increased when the foot is on the ground and the knee is hit on the lateral side and the external rotation torsion is combined with valgus strain force to produce rotary displacement and medial complex rupture [5].

The MPFL is an especially important medial stabilizer, especially for patellofemoral stability. This importance has been demonstrated in various biomechanical knee studies that have shown that the MPFL accounts for more than half of the restraining force that prevents the patella from lateral dislocation [38–40]. Surgical and imaging studies have documented MPFL disruption in approximately 90% to 100% of the patients [41–43]. The identification of MPFL disruption is important; several authors have advocated for the repair of the MPFL when it is present after a patellar dislocation [42,44].

The injury to the MPFL is commonly at or near the femoral origin. This region is well visualized at a discrete anatomic structure on MR imaging, as are associated bone marrow contusion injuries

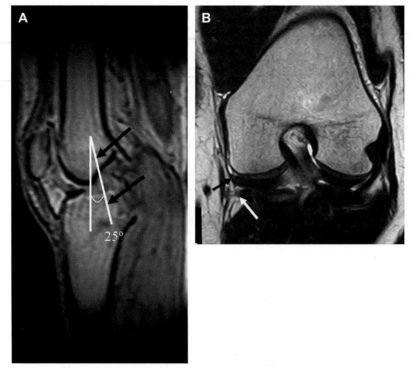

Fig. 25. (A) Sagittal gradient echo localizer MR image of the knee shows the orientation of the scan plane for the coronal oblique sequence obtained for optimal evaluation of the POL. The coronal oblique plane is oriented 25 degrees oblique to a direct coronal (scan plane indicated by *black arrows*). (B) Coronal T2–weighted image without fat saturation shows the POL and its attachment to the medial meniscus (*black arrow*) and the semimembranosis (*white arrow*).

(of the lateral femoral condyle and medial patella) that are commonly seen with lateral patellar dislocation (Fig. 27). The MPFL is consistently visible on axial MR images but it is occasionally ill defined due to partial-volume averaging through an obliquely orientated ligament [45].

There will commonly be other injuries to the medial ligamentous structures, such as tearing of

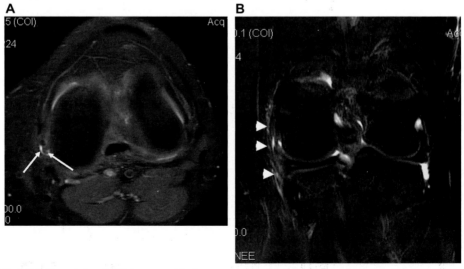

Fig. 26. (A) Axial T2–weighted MR image with fat saturation shows fluid surrounding the POL (*white arrows*). (B) Coronal T2–weighted MR image with fat saturation demonstrates fluid surrounding the posterior oblique ligament (*white arrowheads*).

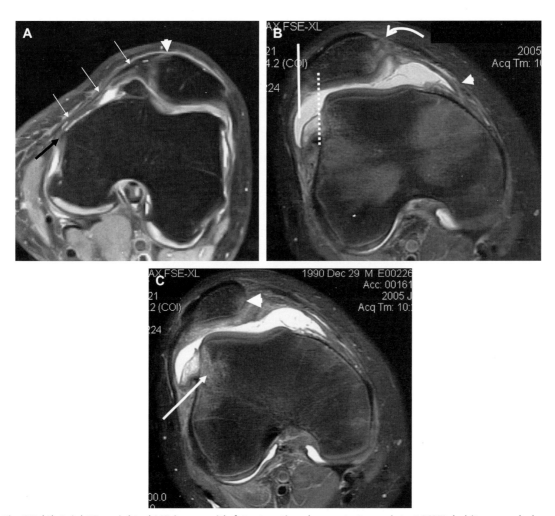

Fig. 27. (A) Axial T2–weighted MR image with fat saturation demonstrates an intact MPFL (*white arrows*) along with its femoral origin (*black arrow*) and its attachment to the superior portion of the patella (*white arrowhead*). (B) Axial T2–weighted MR image with fat saturation in a different patient shows disruption of the MPFL distally (*curved white arrow*) and proximally (*white arrowhead*). There is also lateral displacement of the patella as is evidenced by the location of the lateral border of the patella (*solid white line*) relative to the lateral border of the lateral femoral condyle (*dotted white line*). (C) Axial T2–weighted MR image with fat saturation demonstrates the bone marrow contusion pattern that is typically following a lateral dislocation of the patella with edema along the lateral portion of the lateral femoral condyle (*white arrow*) and the medial portion of the patella (*white arrowhead*).

the medial patellar retinaculum, tearing of the MCL, or stripping of the vastus medialis from its attachment to the adductor tubercle (with or without retraction of the vastus medialis) [46,47]. A large knee joint effusion is also commonly associated with a lateral patellar dislocation and is easily detected on MR imaging.

Osseous MR imaging findings of lateral patellar dislocation may persist after healing of the soft tissue structures and may be indicative of prior lateral patellar dislocation. These findings include osteochondral injuries of the lateral femoral condyle or a concave impaction deformity at the inferomedial patella [46]. Detection of these osseous abnormalities should prompt close scrutiny of the medial ligamentous supporting structures that may have been injured at the time of the lateral patellar dislocation.

Valgus stress with external rotation of the knee may also produce an injury known as the reverse Segond fracture [48]. This fracture involves the medial tibial plateau and is associated with tears of the medial meniscus and the posterior cruciate ligament. As with the Segond fracture, the reverse Segond fracture is well demonstrated on coronal MR images. The fracture is most conspicuous on the coronal T1-weighted images, and the edema associated with the fracture is best noted on the coronal or axial fluid sensitive sequences.

A complete MR imaging evaluation of the knee may also demonstrate thickening of the medial patellar plica. The medial plica arises from the medial capsule of the knee joint, runs inferiorly and obliquely in, and inserts into the synovium covering the infrapatellar fat pad. The thickened medial plica can cause irritation or damage to the anteromedial knee joint by impinging on the articular cartilage of the medial patellar facet in flexion or the cartilage of the medial femoral condyle when the knee is in extension [49]. Axial and sagittal T2-weighted MR images obtained with or without fat saturation are excellent in terms of visualizing the medial patellar plicae. The medial patellar plica has decreased signal intensity on both the T1- and the T2-weighted images. The medial plica is also well defined with some degree of fluid distension within the joint. Although size and shape of the medial plica do not provide firm evidence that the plica is clinically significant, symptomatic plicae are usually thickened and may cause erosion of the medial femoral condyle and patellar cartilage.

Summary

The anatomic supporting structures of the medial and lateral portions of the knee are important components for proper knee function and stability and have long been of interest to the orthopedic and radiology communities and to anatomists. The normal anatomy is interdependent and comprises complex functional structures. Injuries to the normal anatomy may be divided into quadrants (anteromedial, anterolateral, posteromedial, and posterolateral) based on the location of the injury. This division allows for analogous grouping of most of the common injury mechanisms.

The anatomy of the posterolateral corner of the knee is complex and contains the LCL as the major stabilizing structure. Almost all injuries of the LCS are associated with injuries to other posterolateral corner structures. The AOB joins the posterolateral corner with the anterolateral knee structures.

Posterolateral corner injuries are less common than medial knee injuries but usually result from external tibial rotation, posterolaterally directed impact, or from hyperextension. A posterolateral corner injury may be difficult to detect clinically, and an unrepaired injury in this region can lead to chronic posterolateral rotational instability. Radiographs may demonstrate an arcuate sign indicative of a posterolateral corner injury, but this region is best evaluated with MR imaging. The MR evaluation is effective for the ligamentous and tendinous components of the posterolateral corner.

The most important component of the anterolateral knee is the ITT. The AOB functions to distribute force to the anterior and posterior components of the lateral knee, and there is a broad insertion of ITT fibers that attach to the lateral tibia posterior to Gerdy's tubercle.

Injuries to the structures of the anterolateral knee typically occur after a varus blow combined with forceful internal rotation and are commonly associated with tears of the ACL. The most common injured structure of the anterolateral knee is the ITT. This can be associated with a Segond avulsion fracture of the anterolateral tibial rim. Imaging evaluation typically includes conventional radiography, which will readily demonstrate a Segond fracture, but evaluation with MR imaging is effective at evaluating other associated soft tissue injuries (including ACL tears).

The main stabilizer of the posteromedial corner is the MCL. The early anatomic description of the knee that divided the anatomic structures into three layers (crural, superficial ligament, and capsular layers) is still used. The POL is another important component of the posteromedial knee, and this structure is responsible for resistance to valgus stress when the knee is in full extension.

Injuries to the posteromedial knee usually result from a blow to the lateral aspect of the knee or proximal tibia along with external rotation but may also result from twisting injuries without contact. The POL is necessary for knee stability in extension and is functionally independent of the MCL. Injuries to the medial knee are typically classified as first- through third-degree sprain/tear injuries. Although there is often overestimation if the degree of the MCL system with this classification system, it is helpful with third-degree MCL tears because the ligamentous disruption is usually obvious on the MR imaging examination. There may be other associated injuries in the region including injuries to the ACL, the medial meniscus, the POL, the vastus medialis, the semimembranosis, and so forth.

The MR imaging examination best demonstrates injuries to the posteromedial knee on the coronal and axial images, and the medial meniscus should be closely evaluated for extrusion, because higher-grade MCL tears are often associated with medial displacement of the meniscus. The location of an MCL tear is also important to note, because this may have an affect on how the tear is treated. The MR imaging evaluation of the POL is similar to the MCL, but the POL may be better visualized with a coronal oblique plane. The location and extent of injury to the POL may also affect how a tear of this structure is treated.

The MCL, along with the MPFL, is the primary stabilizer of the anteromedial knee. Medial patellar plicae are also seen in this region but do not play an important role in providing stability to the anteromedial knee. The ACL and the medial meniscus are also important anteromedial stabilizers. External rotation, valgus tension, and flexion forces are the typical biomechanical stress that will cause injury to this region.

Disruption of the MPFL can give rise to lateral patellar dislocation and is often associated with MCL tears, a large knee joint effusion, and bone marrow contusions along the medial patella and lateral portion of the lateral femoral condyle. An injury to the MPFL should prompt the investigation for other associated abnormalities.

Valgus stress may also produce a fracture of the medial tibial plateau known as a reverse Segond fracture. This fracture is associated with tears of the medial meniscus and the posterior cruciate ligament. The MR imaging examination typically shows abnormalities of the anteromedial knee most optimally on the axial and coronal images. Fractures are most conspicuous on the T1-weighted images and edema is best seen on the fluid sensitive sequences.

The medial patellar plica is a structure that is normally seen in the anteromedial knee but may become thickened and cause damage to the articular cartilage of the medial patellar facet or the medial femoral condyle. This process is best seen on the fluid sensitive axial MR images of the knee.

Injuries to the lateral and medial supporting structures of the knee can be significantly disabling and can be somewhat difficult to detect and evaluate clinically. An accurate imaging evaluation of these structures requires the use of the appropriate MR imaging sequences and the detailed knowledge of the anatomic structures that are present in these locations. Normal function is dependent on the integrity of the complex functional structures and effective clinical treatment, including surgical repair, of these structures is predicated on an optimal diagnostic evaluation. A successful diagnostic evaluation can expedite treatment and provide the best opportunity for a favorable long-term outcome.

References

[1] Warren LF, Marshall JL. The supporting structures and layers on the medial side of the knee: an anatomical analysis. J Bone Joint Surg Am 1979;61: 56–62.

[2] Seebacher JR, Inglis AE, Marshall JL, et al. The structure of the posterolateral aspect of the knee. J Bone Joint Surg Am 1982;64:536–41.

[3] Hughston JC, Jacobson KE. Chronic posterolateral rotatory instability of the knee. J Bone Joint Surg Am 1985;67:351–9.

[4] Norwood LA, Andrews JR, Meisterling RC, et al. Acute anterolateral rotatory instability of the knee. J Bone Joint Surg Am 1979;61:704–9.

[5] Hughston JC, Barrett GR. Acute anteromedial rotatory instability. Long-term results of surgical repair. J Bone Joint Surg Am 1983;65: 145–53.

[6] Loredo R, Hodler J, Pedowitz R, et al. Posteromedial corner of the knee: MR imaging with gross anatomic correlation. Skeletal Radiol 1999;28: 305–11.

[7] Munshi M, Pretterklieber ML, Kwak S, et al. MR imaging, MR arthrography, and specimen correlation of the posterolateral corner of the knee: an anatomic study. AJR Am J Roentgenol 2003; 180:1095–101.

[8] Fanelli GC, Harris JD. Surgical treatment of acute medial collateral ligament and posteromedial corner injuries of the knee. Sports Med Arthrosc 2006;14(2):78–83.

[9] Cooper JM, McAndrews PT, LaPrade RF. Posterolateral corner injuries of the knee: anatomy, diagnosis, and treatment. Sports Med Arthrosc 2006; 14(4):213–20.

[10] Yu JS, Salonen DC, Hodler J, et al. Posterolateral aspect of the knee: improved MR imaging with a coronal oblique technique. Radiology 1996; 198:199–204.

[11] Haims AH, Medvecky MJ, Pavlovich R Jr, et al. MR imaging of the anatomy of and injuries to the lateral and posterolateral aspects of the knee. Am J Roentgenol 2003;180:647–53.

[12] Campos JC, Chung CB, Lektrakul N, et al. Pathogenesis of the Segond fracture: anatomic and MR imaging evidence of an iliotibial tract or anterior oblique band avulsion. Radiology 2001; 219:381–6.

[13] Last RJ. The popliteus muscle and lateral meniscus: with a note on the attachment of the medial meniscus. J Bone Joint Surg Br 1950;32:93–9.

[14] Staubli HU, Birrer S. The popliteus tendon and its fascicles at the popliteal hiatus: gross anatomy and functional arthroscopic evaluation with and without anterior cruciate ligament deficiency. Arthroscopy 1990;6:209–20.

[15] Johnson LL. Lateral capsular ligament complex: anatomical and surgical considerations. Am J Sports Med 1979;7:156–60.

[16] Terry GC, Hughston JC, Norwood LA. The anatomy of the iliopatellar band and iliotibial tract. Am J Sports Med 1986;14:39–45.

[17] Hughston JC, Eilers AF. The role of the posterior oblique ligament in repairs of acute medial (collateral) ligament tears of the knee. J Bone Joint Surg Am 1973;55:923–39.

[18] Sakakibara J. Arthroscopic study on Iino's band (plica synovialis mediopatellaris). Journal of the Japanese Orthopedic Association 1974;50: 513–22.

[19] Veltri DM, Deng XH, Torzilli PA, et al. The role of the cruciate and posterolateral ligaments in stability of the knee: a biomechanical study. Am J Sports Med 1995;23:436–43.

[20] O'Brien S, Warren RF, Pavlov H, et al. Reconstruction of the chronically insufficient anterior cruciate ligament with the central third of the patellar ligament. J Bone Joint Surg Am 1991; 73:278–86.

[21] Lee J, Papakonstantinou O, Brookenthal KR, et al. Arcuate sign of posterolateral knee injuries: anatomic, radiographic, and MR imaging data related to patterns of injury. Skeletal Radiol 2003;32:619–27.

[22] Shindell R, Walsh WM, Connolly JF. Avulsion fracture of the fibula: the "arcuate sign" of posterolateral knee instability. Nebr Med J 1984; 69(11):369–71.

[23] Arthur A, De Smet AA, Asinger DA, et al. Abnormal superior popliteomeniscal fascicle and posterior pericapsular edema: indirect MR imaging signs of a lateral meniscal tear. AJR Am J Roentgenol 2001;176:63–6.

[24] Mirkopulos N, Myer TJ. Isolated avulsion of the popliteus tendon: a case report. Am J Sports Med 1991;19:417–9.

[25] Westrich GH, Hannafin JA, Potter HG. Isolated rupture and repair of the popliteus tendon. Arthroscopy 1995;11:628–32.

[26] Irizarry JM, Recht MP. MR imaging of knee ligament injuries. In: Karasick D, Schweitzer ME, editors. Seminars in musculoskeletal radiology, vol 1. New York: Thieme Medical; 1997. p. 83–104.

[27] Schweitzer ME, Tran D, Deely DM, et al. Medial collateral ligament injuries: evaluation of multiple signs, prevalence and location of associated bone bruises, and assessment with MR imaging. Radiology 1995;194:825–9.

[28] Brown TR, Quinn SF, Wensel JP, et al. Diagnosis of popliteus injuries with MR imaging. Skeletal Radiol 1995;24:511–4.

[29] Irvine GB, Dias JJ, Finlay DB. Segond fractures of the lateral tibial condyle: brief report. J Bone Joint Surg Br 1987;69:613–4.

[30] Dietz GW, Wilcox DM, Montgomery JB. Segond tibial condyle fracture: lateral capsular ligament avulsion. Radiology 1986;159:467–9.

[31] Goldman AB, Pavlov H, Rubenstein D. The Segond fracture of the lateral tibia: a small avulsion that reflects major ligamentous damage. AJR Am J Roentgenol 1988;151:1163–7.

[32] El-Khoury GY, Daniel WW, Kathol MH. Acute and chronic avulsive injuries. Radiol Clin North Am 1997;35:747–66.

[33] Lerer DB, Umans HR, Hu MX, et al. The role of meniscal root pathology and radial tear in medial meniscal extrusion. Skeletal Radiol 2004;33:569–74.

[34] Boxheimer L, Lutz AM, Zanetti M, et al. Characteristics of displaceable and nondisplaceable meniscal tears at kinematic MR imaging of the knee. Radiology 2006;238(1):221–31.

[35] Azar FM. Evaluation and treatment of chronic medial collateral ligament injuries of the knee. Sports Med Arthrosc 2006;14(2):84–90.

[36] Woo SL, Vogrin TM, Abramowich SD. Healing and repair of ligament injuries in the knee. J Am Acad Orthop Surg 2000;8(6):364–72.

[37] Liu YK, Tipton CM, Matthes RD, et al. An in situ study of the influence of a sclerosing solution in rabbit medial collateral ligaments and its junction strength. Connect Tissue Res 1983; 11(2–3):95–102.

[38] Sandmeier RH, Burks RT, Bachus KN, et al. The effect of reconstruction of the medial patellofemoral ligament on patellar tracking. Am J Sports Med 2000;28:345–9.

[39] Conlan T, Garth WPJ, Lemons JE. Evaluation of the medial soft tissue restraints of the extensor mechanism of the knee. J Bone Joint Surg Am 1993;75:682–93.

[40] Desio SM, Burks RT, Bachus KN. Soft tissue restraints to lateral patellar translation in the human knee. Am J Sports Med 1998;26:59–65.

[41] Spritzer CE, Courneya DL, Burk DLJ, et al. Medial retinacular complex injury in acute patellar dislocation: MR findings and surgical implications. AJR Am J Roentgenol 1997;168: 117–22.

[42] Sallay PI, Poggi J, Speer KP, et al. Acute dislocation of the patella: a correlative pathoanatomic study. Am J Sports Med 1996;24:52–60.

[43] Nomura E. Classification of lesions of the medial patello-femoral ligament in patellar dislocation. Int Orthop 1999;23:260–3.

[44] Muneta T, Sekiya I, Tsuchiya M, et al. A technique for reconstruction of the medial patello-femoral ligament. Clin Orthop 1999;359: 151–5.

[45] Sanders TG, Medynski MA, Feller JF, et al. Bone contusion patterns of the knee at MR imaging: footprint of the mechanism of injury. Radiographics 2000;20:S135–51.

[46] Elias DA, White LM, Fithian DC. Acute lateral patellar dislocation at MR imaging: injury patterns of medial patellar soft-tissue restraints and osteochondral injuries of the inferomedial patella. Radiology 2002;225(3):736–43.

[47] Hunter SC, Marascalco R, Hughston JC. Disruption of the vastus medialis obliquus with medial knee ligament injuries. Am J Sports Med 1983; 11:427–31.

[48] Hall F, Hochman M. Medial Segond-type fracture: cortical avulsion off the medial tibial plateau associated with tears of the posterior cruciate ligament and medial meniscus. Skeletal Radiol 1997;26:553–5.

[49] Garci'a-Valtuille R, Abascal F, Cerezal L, et al. Anatomy and MR imaging appearances of synovial plicae of the knee. Radiographics 2002;22: 775–84.

ELSEVIER
SAUNDERS

RADIOLOGIC
CLINICS
OF NORTH AMERICA

Radiol Clin N Am 45 (2007) 1003–1016

Advanced MR Imaging of the Cruciate Ligaments

Catherine C. Roberts, MD[a],*, Jeffrey D. Towers, MD[b],
Mark J. Spangehl, MD[c], John A. Carrino, MD, MPH[d],
William B. Morrison, MD[e]

- Normal anatomy and sectional appearance
  Anterior cruciate ligament
  Posterior cruciate ligament
- Anterior cruciate ligament acute injury
  Typical tears
  Associated injuries and findings
  Atypical tears and pitfalls
  Anterior cruciate ligament chronic injury
- Posterior cruciate ligament acute injury
  Typical tears and associated injuries
  Atypical tears and pitfalls

- Posterior cruciate ligament chronic injury
- Anterior cruciate ligament reconstruction
  Single-bundle/double-bundle technique
  Evaluation of fixation and graft
  Complications
  Associated findings and mimics of graft failure
- Posterior cruciate ligament reconstruction
  Appearance and failure
  Complications
- Summary
- References

The anterior cruciate ligament (ACL) and the posterior cruciate ligament (PCL) are essential to knee stability and movement. These ligaments are named by the location of their tibial attachments. Each ligament is composed of separate functional bundles that differ in size but are equally important in function. MR imaging best delineates these structures in the acutely injured, chronically injured, and reconstructed states.

Normal anatomy and sectional appearance

Anterior cruciate ligament

The ACL extends from the posteromedial aspect of the lateral femoral condyle to the anteromedial tibial plateau, just anterior to the intercondylar eminence [1]. The femoral attachment is not at the intercondylar notch [1,2], which is a common misconception. On axial images it can be seen reliably

This article was originally published in *Magnetic Resonance Imaging Clinics of North America* 15:1, February 2007.
[a] Department of Radiology, Mayo Clinic College of Medicine, 13400 East Shea Boulevard, Scottsdale, AZ 85259, USA
[b] Division of Musculoskeletal Imaging, Department of Radiology, University of Pittsburgh Medical Center, 200 Lothrop Street, Pittsburgh, PA 15213, USA
[c] Department of Orthopedic Surgery, Mayo Clinic College of Medicine, 13400 East Shea Boulevard, Scottsdale, AZ 85259, USA
[d] Russell H. Morgan Department of Radiology and Radiological Science, Johns Hopkins University School of Medicine, 601 North Caroline Street, JHOC 5165, Baltimore, MD 21287, USA
[e] Thomas Jefferson University Hospital, 132 South 10th Street, Suite 1079a, Philadelphia, PA 19107, USA
* Corresponding author.
E-mail address: roberts.catherine@mayo.edu (C.C. Roberts).

doi:10.1016/j.rcl.2007.08.007

on the first image in which the femoral articular cartilage is seen (Fig. 1). The ligament is intra-articular but extra-synovial [2]. The ACL is significantly smaller in women, with respect to measurements of volume, mass, area, and length [3,4]. The apparent difference between men and women, with regard to ACL size and body weight, and intercondylar notch size, is a controversial topic [3,5].

The ACL can be divided into anteromedial bundles (AMB) and posterolateral bundles (PLB) based on function, although there is no histologic separation [2,6]. The bundles are named by their relative attachment sites on the tibia. The AMB restrains anterior tibial translation relative to the femur, whereas the PLB restrains rotation in near full extension [7]. The AMB rotates laterally around the PLB during knee flexion [2]. Distal fibers of the ACL may extend to the anterior and posterior horns of the lateral meniscus [1,2]. An anatomic variant, consisting of a deltoid-shaped tibial attachment extending the length of the transverse meniscal ligament in the coronal plane, can predispose to impingement and synovitis [8].

On MR imaging, the ACL is seen as an obliquely oriented band of low T1- and T2-weighted signal lying within the lateral aspect of the intercondylar notch. On sagittal images with the knee extended, the ACL bundles are relatively parallel [2]. The PLB is taut, whereas the AMB is slack [1,7]. Imaging the knee with a mild degree of flexion, specifically 30 degrees in one study [9], has been shown to decrease volume averaging in the region of the intercondylar notch, and thus better delineate the ACL. The straight anterior border of the ACL should nearly parallel the Blumensaat line (roof of the intercondylar notch) [10,11].

Posterior cruciate ligament

The PCL is larger and stronger than the ACL [12] and functions to restrain posterior tibial translation relative to the femur [12]. The femoral attachment is along the medial side and medial roof of the intercondylar notch. The tibial attachment is along the midline dorsal aspect of the tibial plateau, between the meniscal roots. The PCL tibial attachment also extends over the dorsal rim of the posterior tibial shelf. The PCL can be divided into two functional bundles, the anterolateral bundle (ALB) and the posteromedial bundle (PMB) [12]. The bundles are named based on the location of their femoral attachments. The two bundles maintain their anterior and posterior locations during motion of the knee and do not rotate around each other [12], as is seen with the bundles of the ACL. The ALB is larger and stronger, but has a co-dominant role with the PMB in stabilizing the knee [13]. Additional posterior oblique fibers of the PCL have been described and can be confused with the posterior meniscofemoral ligament [12]. The meniscofemoral ligaments extend from the posterior horn of the lateral meniscus to the medial femoral condyle. The meniscofemoral ligament lying posterior to the PCL is also known as the ligament of Wrisberg. The meniscofemoral ligament lying anterior to the PCL is also known as the ligament of Humphrey and may mimic an intact PCL in the presence of a PCL tear.

On MR imaging with the knee in an extended position, the normal PCL is seen as a broad band of low T1- and T2-weighted signal, near the midline of the knee, extending from the femoral intercondylar notch to the posterior tibial plateau. On sagittal images with the knee extended, the PCL has a gently

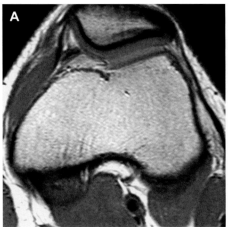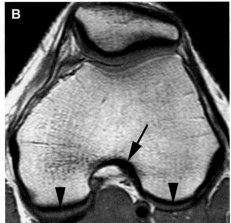

Fig. 1. Normal femoral attachment of the ACL on proton density MR imaging. (*A*) Axial section above common level of ACL origin and femoral articular cartilage. (*B*) Axial level of ACL attachment (*arrow*) and femoral articular cartilage (*arrowheads*).

curved configuration. Although the PCL is slack in the fully extended position, the PMB is relatively taut, compared with the ALB [12]. The PCL shares function with the posterolateral corner structures in providing posterolateral rotatory stability. In flexion it becomes more taut and functional as the posterolateral corner structures become progressively lax (Fig. 2).

A normal joint recess is located just posterior to the PCL, termed the PCL recess. This joint recess communicates with the medial femorotibial compartment and potentially can become isolated from the rest of the joint [14]. An additional small joint recess lies between the ACL and PCL, termed the intercruciate recess [14]. The intercruciate recess may communicate with either the medial or lateral femorotibial compartment [14].

Anterior cruciate ligament acute injury

Typical tears

The ACL should be examined in sagittal, coronal, and axial planes for abnormal increased T2-weighted signal or abnormal contour. An oblique coronal plane, prescribed along the line of the ACL in the sagittal plane, may be of help in low-grade or chronic injuries, or to evaluate the reconstructed ACL (Fig. 3). Signs of a tear include discontinuous fibers, nonvisible fibers, and abnormal slope of the ligament. The sagittal plane (Fig. 4) is most helpful for evaluation of the linear configuration of the ACL fibers [11]. Axial (Fig. 5) and coronal images can confirm findings seen on sagittal images. An oblique sagittal imaging plane can be plotted through the intercondylar notch region and oriented along the course of the ACL. This additional sequence is plotted best using a coronal localizing sequence [15]. Either a conventional spin-echo or a fast spin-echo technique can be used. Fluid-sensitive sequences, including T2-weighted and proton density sequences, are the most sensitive for injury evaluation of the ACL and surrounding soft tissues. T1-weighted and gradient echo sequences are useful to assess for additional injuries in the bones and cartilage.

Tears range from low grade, partial thickness to full thickness and are located most commonly in the mid- to proximal aspect of the ligament. ACL tears occur up to eight times more commonly in females than in males [10,16,17]. A torn ACL fiber has increased T2-weighted signal and an abnormal contour. In some full-thickness tears, an amorphous mass replaces the discrete ACL fibers. Fluid can fill the gap between the fibers of a full-thickness tear (Fig. 6). The location of the tear can be described as proximal (Fig. 7), midsubstance, distal, or involving the femoral or tibial attachment. Women are more likely to have tears involving the proximal ACL, likely because of the higher incidence of noncontact inciting mechanisms [17–19]. If the ACL is torn partially, most commonly the AMB is involved. Avulsion of the ACL from the tibial attachment site is more common in young patients [20].

Associated injuries and findings

Associated injuries and findings include bone bruises, fractures, meniscal tears, anterior subluxation of the tibia, and other ligament injuries. Bone bruises typically are seen at the midlateral femoral condyle and posterior lateral tibial plateau (Fig. 8), although the location can vary, based on injury mechanism [21]. Women are more likely than men to have a posterolateral bone bruise of

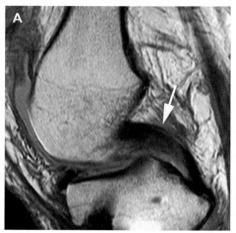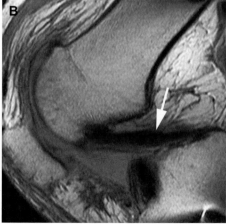

Fig. 2. Normal PCL on sagittal proton density MR imaging in extension and flexion. (*A*) Extension. PCL (*arrow*) is bowed normally, reflecting its laxity as the posterolateral corner is taut. (*B*) Flexion (*arrow*). PCL is taut and provides most posterolateral rotatory stability when posterolateral corner structures are lax.

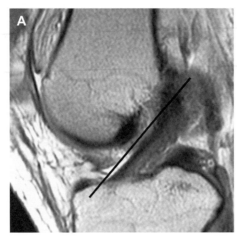
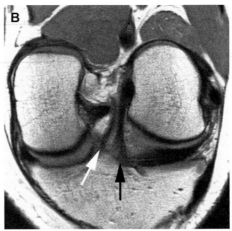

Fig. 3. Normal ACL bundle anatomy on oblique coronal plane. (*A*) Prescription plane (*line*) determined on sagittal T2-weighted image. (*B*) Resultant oblique coronal plane demonstrating ACL AMB (*white arrow*) and ACL PLB (*black arrow*).

the tibia [17]. An impaction fracture along the lateral femoral condyle, referred to as the "deep sulcus sign" (Fig. 9), typically measures more than 2 mm in depth before being a significant indicator of ACL tear. A Segond fracture is an avulsion fracture involving the lateral tibial rim. Classically, this injury was felt to represent an avulsion of the middle third of the lateral capsular ligament. The structure actually avulsed is under debate, and the injury may reflect avulsion of the iliotibial tract and anterior oblique band of the fibular collateral ligament [22]. Usually, meniscal tears are located within the posterior horn of either the medial or lateral meniscus. Additional associated soft tissue injuries include damage to the medial collateral ligament (Fig. 10) and posterolateral corner structures.

Without the stability provided by the ACL, the tibia can sublux anteriorly with respect to the femur (Fig. 11), causing the "anterior tibial translocation sign" [23]. More than 5 to 7 mm of anterior translocation has a high association with an ACL tear [24,25]. The anterior translocation of the tibia can cause the posterior horn of the lateral meniscus to be uncovered, and may also cause the PCL to buckle (Fig. 12). However, a buckled or J-shaped PCL can be seen with or without an ACL tear. Contour abnormalities of the normal PCL can be exaggerated if the patient is imaged in a hyperextended position [26].

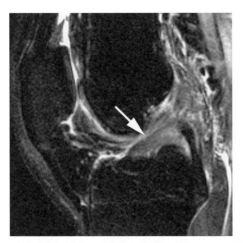

Fig. 4. Partial-thickness tear of the ACL on sagittal fat-suppressed proton density MR imaging. The ACL (*arrow*) has diffusely increased signal. The normal parallel course of the fibers is disrupted. The ACL also has an abnormally horizontal orientation.

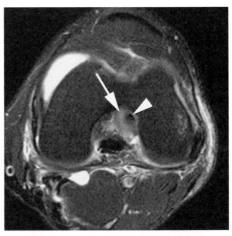

Fig. 5. Partial-thickness ACL tear on corresponding axial T2-weighted MR imaging in same patient as in Fig. 4. Increased signal within the ACL AMB (*arrow*) with residual intact fibers indicates partial-thickness tearing. The adjacent PLB (*arrowhead*) has normal low signal intensity.

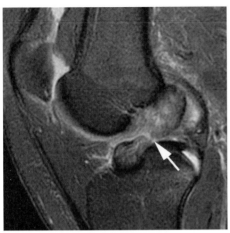

Fig. 6. Full-thickness tear of the ACL on sagittal fat-suppressed T2-weighted MR imaging. Fluid fills the tear (*arrow*) in the midportion of the ligament.

Atypical tears and pitfalls

Rarely, the stump of a full-thickness ACL tear can become entrapped between the femoral condyle and tibial plateau, preventing full extension of the knee [27,28]. These stumps have been characterized as having two appearances: a bulbous stump simulating a Cyclops lesion and a tonguelike stump with focal anterior angulation [27].

Evaluating the ACL for injury has several potential pitfalls. A common pitfall of ACL imaging is volume averaging of the ligament with other structures in the intercondylar notch, including adjacent fluid, fat, and bone. Close examination of the ligament in multiple planes can avoid this pitfall. Fibers of the

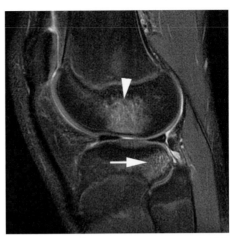

Fig. 8. Bone contusions caused by partial-thickness ACL tear on sagittal fat-suppressed proton density MR imaging. High signal in the lateral femoral condyle (*arrowhead*) and posterior aspect of the lateral tibial plateau (*arrow*) are typical for the "kissing contusions" caused by a pivot shift knee injury.

ACL may be separated by thin lines of fat distally, so this should also not be confused with injury. The ACL can undergo mucoid degeneration, mimicking a tear because of increased T2-weighted signal of the ligament fibers [29,30]. Degeneration, however, would not be associated with any secondary signs of injury. Another cause of high signal within the ACL is the development of a ganglion cyst. The cause is unknown, but has been associated with prior trauma [31,32]. These high T2-weighted signal cysts displace the normal tendon fibers and can be confused with an ACL tear. Ganglia and

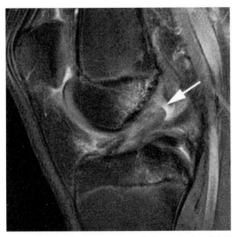

Fig. 7. Near full-thickness tear of the proximal ACL on fat-suppressed proton density MR imaging. The proximal ACL (*arrow*) is seen as a stump of intermediate signal. A few of the anterior superior fibers may remain attached.

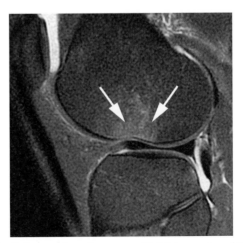

Fig. 9. Deep sulcus sign on sagittal fat-suppressed T2-weighted MR imaging. An impaction fracture of the lateral femoral condyle with surrounding edema (*arrows*) was associated with a partial-thickness ACL tear.

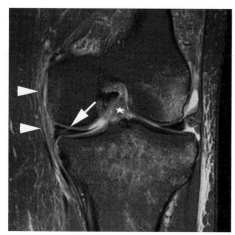

Fig. 10. High-grade partial-thickness ACL tear (*) on coronal fat-suppressed T2-weighted MR imaging. Associated findings include medial collateral ligament tear (*arrowheads*), medial meniscus posterior horn tear (*arrow*), and multifocal bone contusions.

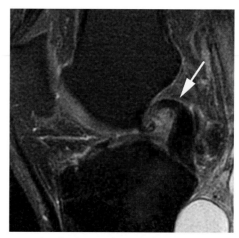

Fig. 12. A hooked, or J-shaped, PCL (*arrow*) is associated with a full-thickness ACL tear (not shown) on sagittal fat-suppressed proton density MR imaging.

mucoid degeneration can coexist and are unrelated to instability [33]. A final pitfall is that the ACL may be hypoplastic or absent, as a normal variant [34–36].

Anterior cruciate ligament chronic injury

With conservative therapy, partial and complete ACL tears can regain continuity [37,38]. The healing process of the ACL includes the formation of scar tissue that is weaker than the original ligament fibers [39]. As the ACL heals, the increased T2-signal

begins to resolve on MR imaging. Scar tissue can cause the ligament fibers to become thickened and indistinct, or the scar tissue can mask the signs of prior injury entirely [40]. The ACL may form bridging scar tissue to the region of the intercondylar notch (Fig. 13) or PCL.

Patients who have ACL-deficient knees may show abnormal anterior tibial subluxation [41], which can worsen over time [42]. Although the ACL functions to restrain rotation, significant alterations in tibial rotation were not documented on a recent study evaluating ACL-deficient knees with MR imaging [41].

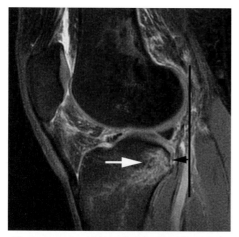

Fig. 11. Anteriorly subluxed tibia (*black arrow*) with respect to the posterior aspect of the femoral condyle (*line*) on sagittal fat-suppressed proton density MR imaging. A full-thickness ACL tear was present. A bone contusion (*white arrow*) is located in the posterior aspect of the lateral tibial plateau.

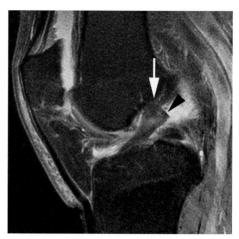

Fig. 13. Chronic full-thickness ACL tear on sagittal fat-suppressed proton density MR imaging. The torn ACL (*arrowhead*) has adhered partially to the intercondylar notch roof (*arrow*).

Posterior cruciate ligament acute injury

Typical tears and associated injuries

The PCL is injured less commonly than the ACL, but can demonstrate the same range of appearances on MR imaging, from focal areas of abnormal signal to complete disruption of the ligament. The PCL is evaluated best on sagittal MR images obtained with a fluid-sensitive sequence. The PCL most commonly tears at the midportion of the ligament (Fig. 14), and is more likely than the ACL to have a partial tear [43]. Regardless of the imaging modality used, it can be difficult sometimes to differentiate partial- from full-thickness tears [44]. MR classification systems of tears have been proposed but are not used widely [45].

PCL injuries have a high association with other injuries. Trabecular microfractures, or bone bruises, are seen commonly. The reported incidence ranges from 32% to 83% [46,47]. Unlike the bone bruises associated with ACL tears, the bruises associated with PCL tears have a less predictable location, and can be located medially, laterally, or within the patella [47]. Up to one half of PCL tears also have medial collateral ligament and meniscal tears. Full-thickness PCL tears may be associated with posterior translation of the tibia with respect to the femur (Fig. 15) because of the lack of ligamentous support.

PCL tears are associated with posterolateral corner injuries [48]. Attention should be directed to the soft tissues of the lateral and posterolateral aspect of the knee, to exclude this injury pattern. Co-existing posterolateral corner injuries act to worsen knee instability and can accelerate secondary degenerative change.

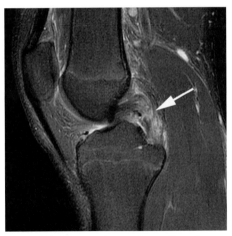

Fig. 15. Full-thickness PCL tear (*arrow*) and posterior subluxation of tibia with respect to femur on sagittal fat-suppressed T2-weighted MR imaging.

Atypical tears and pitfalls

A few unusual variants of PCL injury have been reported in the literature. A "peel-off" PCL tear refers to a full-thickness tear along the femoral attachment, without an avulsion fracture. This tear has an arthroscopic option for repair [49]. An avulsion fracture of the femoral attachment of the PCL has been seen with knee dislocation and popliteal artery rupture in a child [50]. Isolated tears of the PMB can be seen [51] as well. Finally, it is also somewhat unusual to have a PCL tear in the absence of other injuries, such as bone contusions, ligament strain or tear, or meniscal injuries.

Magic angle artifact can produce foci of increased T1-weighted signal within the PCL in the absence of injury or degeneration. The magic angle artifact will occur in any structure, usually a tendon or ligament, oriented 55 degrees to the main magnetic field. Because this MR artifact is limited to sequences with a short echo time, there will be no corresponding abnormal signal on proton density or T2-weighted sequences.

A ruptured PCL rarely can maintain a normal contour [52]. Another potential pitfall is the "double PCL sign" caused by a displaced bucket-handle tear of the medial meniscus (Fig. 16). The displaced meniscal tissue can lie parallel to the PCL on a sagittal image and should not be confused with a PCL injury.

Posterior cruciate ligament chronic injury

As with the ACL, partial- or full-thickness PCL tears may regain continuity of the ligament fibers with only conservative therapy [37]. When a PCL injury consists of a focus of increased T2-weighted signal

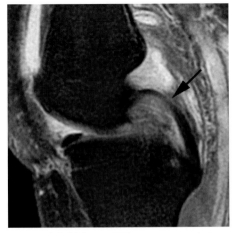

Fig. 14. Partial-thickness PCL tear seen as intermediate signal in the mid- (*arrow*) and proximal portions of the ligament on sagittal fat-suppressed proton density MR imaging.

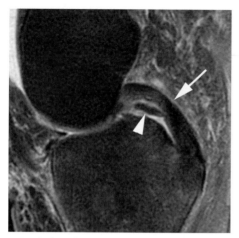

Fig. 16. Displaced meniscal tissue (*arrowhead*) lying adjacent to the PCL (*arrow*) may simulate a PCL injury, seen on sagittal fat-suppressed proton density MR.

within a continuous ligamentous band, conservative therapy can be considered. Patients with this MR appearance have preserved or improving joint stability over time [53,54]. After injury and subsequent healing, the PCL may return to homogeneous, normal, low signal intensity on MR imaging. The chronically injured PCL may be thickened or elongated (Fig. 17).

The PCL-deficient knee may show abnormal posterior subluxation of the tibia with respect to the femur, up to 44% of which cannot be reduced using anterior force [55]. The ACL can be weakened by chronic PCL injury, resulting in decreased diameter, size, and number of collagen fibrils [56].

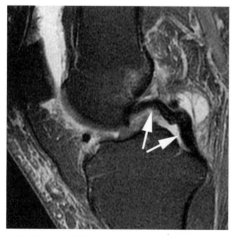

Fig. 17. Chronic PCL tear on sagittal fat-suppressed T2-weighted MR imaging. After partial-thickness tear 3 years prior, the PCL (*arrows*) has healed with an elongated, undulating contour. The tibia is subluxed posteriorly with respect to the femur.

Anterior cruciate ligament reconstruction

The ACL can be reconstructed using various materials and techniques. Autograft tendon, allograft tendon, or synthetic materials may be used. Autograft materials, using the central third of the patellar tendon, with attached bone, or the distal hamstring tendon, are used most widely. The use of synthetic grafts has fallen out of favor because of high complication and failure rates [57]. Reconstruction of the ACL-deficient knee is recommended within 1 year of injury to reduce the incidence of secondary meniscal tears and degenerative change [58,59].

Single-bundle/double-bundle technique

Traditional ACL reconstruction functionally replaces only the AMB of the ACL. The double-bundle technique of ACL repair involves placement of a double ligament, using up to four bone tunnels (Fig. 18) [60]. The goal of this procedure is to restore normal biomechanical function to the knee after ACL injury [61]. The surgical technique used for a double-bundle repair varies, including location of the access portals, type of fixation device, placement of bone tunnels, number and size of tunnels, and intraoperative position of the knee [60]. Allograft and autograft materials can be used. As 3-Tesla MR imaging becomes used more widely in clinical applications, it will facilitate distinguishing the two bundles of the ACL [62], which has future implications for preoperatively determining the extent of injury of each bundle and potentially preserving one of the bundles during reconstruction [62]. Occasionally, a single native bundle and a single reconstructed bundle are seen in a single-bundle reconstruction. Distinguishing this technique from single-bundle reconstruction may be a challenge, but oblique sagittal plane images usually suffice in distinguishing native and graft elements (Fig. 19).

Evaluation of fixation and graft

MR imaging is crucial for evaluating the postoperative knee [63]. The reconstructed or repaired ligament, bone, cartilage, menisci, and surrounding soft tissues all can be evaluated with this modality. The graft should be assessed in oblique sagittal, coronal, and axial planes. T2-weighted MR sequences improve visualization of the graft fibers. MR evaluation of the integrity of an ACL graft can also be enhanced by MR arthrography [64,65]. The intra-articular administration of a dilute gadolinium mixture outlines the course of the graft and can accentuate regions of graft discontinuity. The use of intravenous gadolinium can also be useful in assessing graft morphology [66].

MR signal of the ACL graft varies, based on the composition and age of the graft. In the early

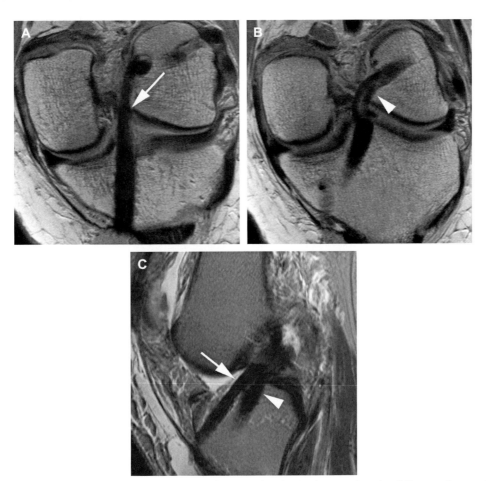

Fig. 18. Double-bundle ACL repair. Oblique coronal proton density MR images showing (*A*) normal reconstructed AMB (*arrow*) and (*B*) PLB (*arrowhead*). (*C*) Oblique sagittal FSE T2-weighted MR image showing AMB (*arrow*) and PLB (*arrowhead*).

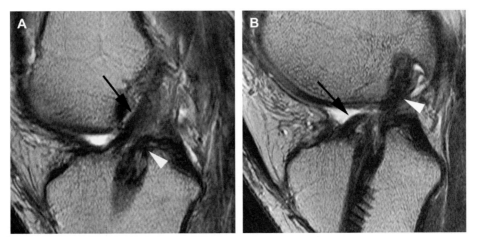

Fig. 19. Single PLB ACL reconstruction. (*A*) Sagittal FSE T2-weighted MR imaging showing native AMB (*arrow*) and posterolateral tibial tunnel (*arrowhead*). (*B*) Adjacent image showing native AMB tibial insertion (*arrow*) and PLB graft in section (*arrowhead*).

postoperative state, grafts are hypovascular and typically have low signal intensity on all sequences. In the late postoperative period, between 4 and 8 months, the graft remodels and may show as focal or diffuse, increased T2-weighted signal [67]. This change in signal is attributed to "ligamentization" of the graft [68]. After 1 year, grafts typically return to their normal low T1- and T2-weighted signal intensity, although persistence of increased signal has been reported beyond the first postoperative year [66].

The normal location of the femoral graft tunnel on sagittal images is at the junction of the intercondylar roof (physeal scar level) and posterior femoral cortex [69]. The femoral tunnel should be seen on coronal MR images in the 11 o'clock position for the right knee and in the 1 o'clock position for the left knee [70]. The tibial tunnel should lie parallel and posterior to the Blumensaat line (Fig. 20), between the anterior tibial tubercle and the posterior border of the tibia near the midline [69]. Graft fixation devices include a myriad of screws (metal and biodegradable), staples, buttons, and bone plugs.

Complications

Complications from ACL repair can be related to graft harvesting, graft placement, or the graft itself. Graft harvesting can result in complications to the donor site. For patellar tendon grafts, the remaining portion of the tendon can rupture, the patella can fracture, or arthrofibrosis can develop, resulting in patella baja. Vascular injuries can occur during graft harvesting, but are uncommon [71].

If a graft is placed incorrectly, other complications can result. A tibial tunnel placed too far anteriorly can result in graft impingement along the intercondylar notch roof. The impinged graft will contact the roof of the intercondylar notch and may appear bowed posteriorly. Increased T2-weighted signal is present in the distal two thirds of the impinged graft. A tibial tunnel placed too far laterally can result in graft impingement along the medial aspect of the lateral femoral condyle [72]. Fixation hardware can fail in several ways, including fracture, loosening, failure of union, and displacement. Placement of the graft can lead to the fracture of the tibia or femur, either during or after ACL repair [73–75]. No complications have been related specifically to the use of the double-bundle reconstruction technique [60], apart from those complications seen with other techniques.

The graft itself can tear or stretch. Tears are seen as intermediate to high T2-weighted signal within the graft, taking into account the normal transition of signal intensity during revascularization and resynovialization of the graft in the 4- to 8-month postoperative period. Thinning and an abnormal contour of the graft fibers indicate tearing (Fig. 21). Partial-thickness tears will have some remaining fibers visible. The stretched graft will appear intact but have an elongated appearance and can have associated signs of graft bucking, anterior tibial subluxation, or uncovering of the lateral meniscus posterior horn.

Arthrofibrosis may develop in the anterior aspect of the knee, producing a decreased range of motion. Focal arthrofibrosis anterior to the distal aspect of the graft is referred to as a "cyclops" lesion

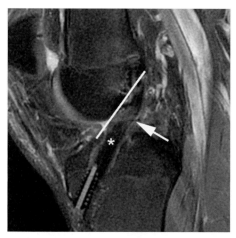

Fig. 20. Normal ACL reconstruction on 5-month follow-up sagittal fat-suppressed proton density MR imaging. Normal graft (*) location is posterior and parallel to Blumensaat line (*line*). Increased signal (*arrow*) in the midportion is normal within the first post operative year.

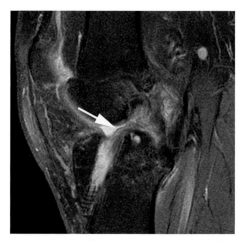

Fig. 21. Rupture of ACL graft on sagittal fat-suppressed proton density MR imaging. Graft fibers (*arrow*) are markedly thin and have an abnormally horizontal course.

(Fig. 22). Diffuse arthrofibrosis appears as low signal fibrous tissue in Hoffa's fat pad.

Associated findings and mimics of graft failure

Hamstring grafts normally contain linear regions of intermediate signal and fluid because of the graft being composed of multiple bundles. The hamstring graft is composed of a segment of semitendinosus and gracilis tendon doubled back on itself, giving a total of four bundles for increased graft strength, which may simulate a graft tear because the striated appearance and regions of linear fluid would not be seen normally with a patellar tendon graft [69]. The use of hamstring reconstruction has been associated with sclerosis and widening of bone tunnels [76,77], but this is of uncertain clinical significance [60]. An increase in the size of the graft does not indicate pathology necessarily, because the normal patellar tendon graft can hypertrophy after placement [78].

Loose bodies within the joint may limit range of motion and simulate arthrofibrosis. Ganglion cysts can develop within the graft, just as they can develop within the native ACL, and potentially can limit range of motion and simulate a tear. Ganglion cysts within ACL grafts have not been associated definitively with graft failure.

Posterior cruciate ligament reconstruction

Most PCL tears are partial thickness, as opposed to full thickness, and can be treated with conservative therapy. In some cases, the partially torn PCL can be repaired directly. Metal artifact and fibrous tissue can obscure the repair site (Fig. 23). For those injuries needing reconstruction, the materials used are similar to those for ACL reconstruction. Single-bundle or double-bundle reconstruction techniques can be used [79].

Appearance and failure

The normal appearance of the reconstructed PCL is somewhat controversial in the literature. The PCL graft likely undergoes a normal postoperative change in signal intensity similar to ACL grafts [80], although this change is not accepted uniformly. Thickening of the PCL graft is normal in the postoperative period.

PCL graft failure has a similar appearance to ACL graft failure. Intermediate T2-weighted signal within the graft, excluding the 4- to 8-month postoperative period, suggests partial-thickness tearing. Disruption of the graft fibers with interposed fluid signal intensity indicates full-thickness tearing.

Complications

Most PCL reconstruction complications are similar to those of ACL reconstruction. However, arthrofibrosis is present in most patients who have PCL reconstruction [80]. The fibrous tissue can be located anterior or posterior to the graft and may act to improve stability [81].

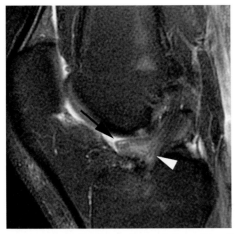

Fig. 22. Cyclops lesion (*arrow*), consisting of localized fibrous tissue on sagittal fat-suppressed T2-weighted MR imaging. Increased signal and an undulating contour of the adjacent ACL graft (*arrowhead*) suggests graft impingement.

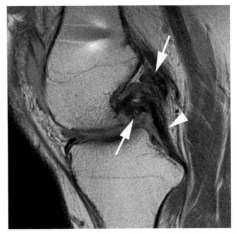

Fig. 23. PCL reconstruction with staple fixation to the distal femur on sagittal proton density MR imaging. The proximal PCL (*between arrows*) is obscured by a nodular mass of mixed low and intermediate signal, most consistent with a partial-thickness tear and prominent chronic fibrotic reactive change. The distal PCL (*arrowhead*) is taut, making a full-thickness tear unlikely.

Summary

MR imaging is accurate and sensitive, making it the study of choice to evaluate the cruciate ligaments of the knee. Acute and chronic injuries can be characterized accurately and differentiated from imaging pitfalls, including artifacts, and anatomic variants. Knowledge of normal ligament reconstruction techniques allows differentiation of the normal postoperative appearance from reconstruction failure and complications.

References

[1] Giron F, Cuomo P, Aglietti P, et al. Femoral attachment of the anterior cruciate ligament. Knee Surg Sports Traumatol Arthrosc 2006; 14(3):250–6.

[2] Duthon VB, Barea C, Abrassart S, et al. Anatomy of the anterior cruciate ligament. Knee Surg Sports Traumatol Arthrosc 2006;14(3):204–13.

[3] Anderson AF, Dome DC, Gautam S, et al. Correlation of anthropometric measurements, strength, anterior cruciate ligament size, and intercondylar notch characteristics to sex differences in anterior cruciate ligament tear rates. Am J Sports Med 2001;29(1):58–66.

[4] Chandrashekar N, Slauterbeck J, Hashemi J. Sex-based differences in the anthropometric characteristics of the anterior cruciate ligament and its relation to intercondylar notch geometry: a cadaveric study. Am J Sports Med 2005;33(10): 1492–8.

[5] Charlton WP, St John TA, Ciccotti MG, et al. Differences in femoral notch anatomy between men and women: a magnetic resonance imaging study. Am J Sports Med 2002;30(3):329–33.

[6] Colombet P, Robinson J, Christel P, et al. Morphology of anterior cruciate ligament attachments for anatomic reconstruction: a cadaveric dissection and radiographic study. Arthroscopy 2006;22(9):984–92.

[7] Petersen W, Zantop T. Anatomy of the anterior cruciate ligament with regard to its two bundles. Clin Orthop Relat Res 2007;454:35–47.

[8] Calpur OU, Ozcan M, Gurbuz H. Deltoid (triangular)-shaped anterior cruciate ligament that caused notch impingement: a report of two cases. Arthroscopy 2004;20(6):637–40.

[9] Lee SY, Matsui N, Yoshida K, et al. Magnetic resonance delineation of the anterior cruciate ligament of the knee: flexed knee position within a surface coil. Clin Imaging 2005;29(2):117–22.

[10] Lee K, Siegel MJ, Lau DM, et al. Anterior cruciate ligament tears: MR imaging-based diagnosis in a pediatric population. Radiology 1999;213(3): 697–704.

[11] Moore SL. Imaging the anterior cruciate ligament. Orthop Clin North Am 2002;33(4): 663–74.

[12] Amis AA, Gupte CM, Bull AM, et al. Anatomy of the posterior cruciate ligament and the meniscofemoral ligaments. Knee Surg Sports Traumatol Arthrosc 2006;14(3):257–63.

[13] Ahmad CS, Cohen ZA, Levine WN, et al. Codominance of the individual posterior cruciate ligament bundles. An analysis of bundle lengths and orientation. Am J Sports Med 2003;31(2): 221–5.

[14] de Abreu MR, Kim HJ, Chung CB, et al. Posterior cruciate ligament recess and normal posterior capsular insertional anatomy: MR imaging of cadaveric knees. Radiology 2005;236(3):968–73.

[15] Barberie JE, Carson BW, Finnegan M, et al. Oblique sagittal view of the anterior cruciate ligament: comparison of coronal vs. axial planes as localizing sequences. J Magn Reson Imaging 2001;14(3):203–6.

[16] Huston LJ, Greenfield ML, Wojtys EM. Anterior cruciate ligament injuries in the female athlete. Potential risk factors. Clin Orthop Relat Res 2000;(372):50–63.

[17] Fayad LM, Parellada JA, Parker L, et al. MR imaging of anterior cruciate ligament tears: is there a gender gap? Skeletal Radiol 2003;32(11): 639–46.

[18] Griffin LY, Agel J, Albohm MJ, et al. Noncontact anterior cruciate ligament injuries: risk factors and prevention strategies. J Am Acad Orthop Surg 2000;8(3):141–50.

[19] Hewett TE, Myer GD, Ford KR. Anterior cruciate ligament injuries in female athletes: Part 1, mechanisms and risk factors. Am J Sports Med 2006;34(2):299–311.

[20] Prince JS, Laor T, Bean JA. MRI of anterior cruciate ligament injuries and associated findings in the pediatric knee: changes with skeletal maturation. AJR Am J Roentgenol 2005;185(3):756–62.

[21] Mohana-Borges AV, Resnick D, Chung CB. Magnetic resonance imaging of knee instability. Semin Musculoskelet Radiol 2005;9(1):17–33.

[22] Campos JC, Chung CB, Lektrakul N, et al. Pathogenesis of the Segond fracture: anatomic and MR imaging evidence of an iliotibial tract or anterior oblique band avulsion. Radiology 2001; 219(2):381–6.

[23] Chiu SS. The anterior tibial translocation sign. Radiology 2006;239(3):914–5.

[24] Gentili A, Seeger LL, Yao L, et al. Anterior cruciate ligament tear: indirect signs at MR imaging. Radiology 1994;193(3):835–40.

[25] Chan WP, Peterfy C, Fritz RC, et al. MR diagnosis of complete tears of the anterior cruciate ligament of the knee: importance of anterior subluxation of the tibia. AJR Am J Roentgenol 1994; 162(2):355–60.

[26] Crotty JM, Monu JU, Pope TL Jr. Magnetic resonance imaging of the musculoskeletal system. Part 4. The knee. Clin Orthop Relat Res 1996;(330):288–303.

[27] Huang GS, Lee CH, Chan WP, et al. Acute anterior cruciate ligament stump entrapment in

anterior cruciate ligament tears: MR imaging appearance. Radiology 2002;225(2):537–40.

[28] Jomha NM, Clingeleffer A, Pinczewski L. Intraarticular mechanical blocks and full extension in patients undergoing anterior cruciate ligament reconstruction. Arthroscopy 2000;16(2):156–9.

[29] McIntyre J, Moelleken S, Tirman P. Mucoid degeneration of the anterior cruciate ligament mistaken for ligamentous tears. Skeletal Radiol 2001;30(6):312–5.

[30] Melloni P, Valls R, Yuguero M, et al. Mucoid degeneration of the anterior cruciate ligament with erosion of the lateral femoral condyle. Skeletal Radiol 2004;33(6):359–62.

[31] Kakutani K, Yoshiya S, Matsui N, et al. An intraligamentous ganglion cyst of the anterior cruciate ligament after a traumatic event. Arthroscopy 2003;19(9):1019–22.

[32] Krudwig WK, Schulte KK, Heinemann C. Intraarticular ganglion cysts of the knee joint: a report of 85 cases and review of the literature. Knee Surg Sports Traumatol Arthrosc 2004;12(2):123–9.

[33] Bergin D, Morrison WB, Carrino JA, et al. Anterior cruciate ligament ganglia and mucoid degeneration: coexistence and clinical correlation. AJR Am J Roentgenol 2004;182(5):1283–7.

[34] Manner HM, Radler C, Ganger R, et al. Dysplasia of the cruciate ligaments: radiographic assessment and classification. J Bone Joint Surg Am 2006;88(1):130–7.

[35] Frikha R, Dahmene J, Ben Hamida R, et al. Absence congenitale du ligament croise anterieur. A propos de 8 cas [Congenital absence of the anterior cruciate ligament: eight cases in the same family]. Rev Chir Orthop Reparatrice Appar Mot 2005;91(7):642–8.

[36] De Ponti A, Sansone V, de Gama Malcher M. Bilateral absence of the anterior cruciate ligament. Arthroscopy 2001;17(6):E26.

[37] Boks SS, Vroegindeweij D, Koes BW, et al. Follow-up of posttraumatic ligamentous and meniscal knee lesions detected at MR imaging: systematic review. Radiology 2006;238(3):863–71.

[38] Fujimoto E, Sumen Y, Ochi M, et al. Spontaneous healing of acute anterior cruciate ligament (ACL) injuries - conservative treatment using an extension block soft brace without anterior stabilization. Arch Orthop Trauma Surg 2002;122(4):212–6.

[39] Frank CB. Ligament structure, physiology and function. J Musculoskelet Neuronal Interact 2004;4(2):199–201.

[40] Vahey TN, Broome DR, Kayes KJ, et al. Acute and chronic tears of the anterior cruciate ligament: differential features at MR imaging. Radiology 1991;181(1):251–3.

[41] Barrance PJ, Williams GN, Snyder-Mackler L, et al. Altered knee kinematics in ACL-deficient non-copers: a comparison using dynamic MRI. J Orthop Res 2006;24(2):132–40.

[42] Mishima S, Takahashi S, Kondo S, et al. Anterior tibial subluxation in anterior cruciate ligament-deficient knees: quantification using magnetic resonance imaging. Arthroscopy 2005;21(10):1193–6.

[43] Sanders TG, Miller MD. A systematic approach to magnetic resonance imaging interpretation of sports medicine injuries of the knee. Am J Sports Med 2005;33(1):131–48.

[44] Miller TT. Sonography of injury of the posterior cruciate ligament of the knee. Skeletal Radiol 2002;31(3):149–54.

[45] Bellelli A, Mancini P, Polito M, et al. Magnetic resonance imaging of posterior cruciate ligament injuries: a new classification of traumatic tears. Radiol Med (Torino) 2006;111(6):828–35.

[46] Sonin AH, Fitzgerald SW, Hoff FL, et al. MR imaging of the posterior cruciate ligament: normal, abnormal, and associated injury patterns. Radiographics 1995;15(3):551–61.

[47] Mair SD, Schlegel TF, Gill TJ, et al. Incidence and location of bone bruises after acute posterior cruciate ligament injury. Am J Sports Med 2004;32(7):1681–7.

[48] Malone AA, Dowd GS, Saifuddin A. Injuries of the posterior cruciate ligament and posterolateral corner of the knee. Injury 2006;37(6):485–501.

[49] Ross G, Driscoll J, McDevitt E, et al. Arthroscopic posterior cruciate ligament repair for acute femoral "peel off" tears. Arthroscopy 2003;19(4):431–5.

[50] Hesse E, Bastian L, Zeichen J, et al. Femoral avulsion fracture of the posterior cruciate ligament in association with a rupture of the popliteal artery in a 9-year-old boy: a case report. Knee Surg Sports Traumatol Arthrosc 2006;14(4):335–9.

[51] Fritz RC. MR imaging of meniscal and cruciate ligament injuries. Magn Reson Imaging Clin N Am 2003;11(2):283–93.

[52] Peterson DC, Thain LM, Fowler PJ. Posterior cruciate ligament imaging. J Knee Surg 2002;15(2):121–7.

[53] Adachi N, Ochi M, Sumen Y, et al. Temporal changes in posterior laxity after isolated posterior cruciate ligament injury: 35 patients examined by stress radiography and MRI. Acta Orthop Scand 2003;74(6):683–8.

[54] Akisue T, Kurosaka M, Yoshiya S, et al. Evaluation of healing of the injured posterior cruciate ligament: analysis of instability and magnetic resonance imaging. Arthroscopy 2001;17(3):264–9.

[55] Strobel MJ, Weiler A, Schulz MS, et al. Fixed posterior subluxation in posterior cruciate ligament-deficient knees: diagnosis and treatment of a new clinical sign. Am J Sports Med 2002;30(1):32–8.

[56] Ochi M, Murao T, Sumen Y, et al. Isolated posterior cruciate ligament insufficiency induces morphological changes of anterior cruciate ligament collagen fibrils. Arthroscopy 1999;15(3):292–6.

[57] Recht MP, Parker RD, Irizarry JM. Second time around: evaluating the postoperative anterior cruciate ligament. Magn Reson Imaging Clin N Am 2000;8(2):285–97.

[58] Faber KJ, Dill JR, Amendola A, et al. Occult osteochondral lesions after anterior cruciate ligament rupture. Six-year magnetic resonance imaging follow-up study. Am J Sports Med 1999;27(4):489–94.

[59] Nelson F, Billinghurst RC, Pidoux I, et al. Early post-traumatic osteoarthritis-like changes in human articular cartilage following rupture of the anterior cruciate ligament. Osteoarthritis Cartilage 2006;14(2):114–9.

[60] Steckel H, Starman JS, Baums MH, et al. The double-bundle technique for anterior cruciate ligament reconstruction: a systematic overview. Scandinavian Journal of Medicine & Science in Sports 2007;17(2):99–108.

[61] Buoncristiani AM, Tjoumakaris FP, Starman JS, et al. Anatomic double-bundle anterior cruciate ligament reconstruction. Arthroscopy 2006; 22(9):1000–6.

[62] Steckel H, Vadala G, Davis D, et al. 2D and 3D 3-tesla magnetic resonance imaging of the double bundle structure in anterior cruciate ligament anatomy. Knee Surg Sports Traumatol Arthrosc 2006;14(11):1151–8.

[63] Ilaslan H, Sundaram M, Miniaci A. Imaging evaluation of the postoperative knee ligaments. Eur J Radiol 2005;54(2):178–88.

[64] McCauley TR, Elfar A, Moore A, et al. MR arthrography of anterior cruciate ligament reconstruction grafts. AJR Am J Roentgenol 2003;181(5):1217–23.

[65] Chung CB, Isaza IL, Angulo M, et al. MR arthrography of the knee: how, why, when. Radiol Clin North Am 2005;43(4):733–46, viii–ix.

[66] Vogl TJ, Schmitt J, Lubrich J, et al. Reconstructed anterior cruciate ligaments using patellar tendon ligament grafts: diagnostic value of contrast-enhanced MRI in a 2-year follow-up regimen. Eur Radiol 2001;11(8):1450–6.

[67] Cheung Y, Magee TH, Rosenberg ZS, et al. MRI of anterior cruciate ligament reconstruction. J Comput Assist Tomogr 1992;16(1):134–7.

[68] Marumo K, Saito M, Yamagishi T, et al. The "ligamentization" process in human anterior cruciate ligament reconstruction with autogenous patellar and hamstring tendons: a biochemical study. Am J Sports Med 2005;33(8):1166–73.

[69] Sanders TG. MR imaging of postoperative ligaments of the knee. Semin Musculoskelet Radiol 2002;6(1):19–33.

[70] Recht MP, Kramer J. MR imaging of the postoperative knee: a pictorial essay. Radiographics 2002; 22(4):765–74.

[71] Milankov M, Miljkovic N, Stankovic M. Pseudoaneurysm of the medial inferior genicular artery following anterior cruciate ligament reconstruction with hamstring tendon autograft. Knee 2006;13(2):170–1.

[72] Papakonstantinou O, Chung CB, Chanchairujira K, et al. Complications of anterior cruciate ligament reconstruction: MR imaging. Eur Radiol 2003;13(5): 1106–17.

[73] Manktelow AR, Haddad FS, Goddard NJ. Late lateral femoral condyle fracture after anterior cruciate ligament reconstruction. A case report. Am J Sports Med 1998;26(4):587–90.

[74] Wilson TC, Rosenblum WJ, Johnson DL. Fracture of the femoral tunnel after an anterior cruciate ligament reconstruction. Arthroscopy 2004; 20(5):e45–7.

[75] Thaunat M, Nourissat G, Gaudin P, et al. Tibial plateau fracture after anterior cruciate ligament reconstruction: role of the interference screw resorption in the stress riser effect. Knee 2006; 13(3):241–3.

[76] Clatworthy MG, Annear P, Bulow JU, et al. Tunnel widening in anterior cruciate ligament reconstruction: a prospective evaluation of hamstring and patella tendon grafts. Knee Surg Sports Traumatol Arthrosc 1999;7(3):138–45.

[77] Jansson KA, Harilainen A, Sandelin J, et al. Bone tunnel enlargement after anterior cruciate ligament reconstruction with the hamstring autograft and endobutton fixation technique. A clinical, radiographic and magnetic resonance imaging study with 2 years follow-up. Knee Surg Sports Traumatol Arthrosc 1999;7(5): 290–5.

[78] Shimizu K, Yoshiya S, Kurosaka M, et al. Change in the cross-sectional area of a patellar tendon graft after anterior cruciate ligament reconstruction. Knee Surg Sports Traumatol Arthrosc 2006; [Epub ahead of print].

[79] Makino A, Aponte Tinao L, Ayerza MA, et al. Anatomic double-bundle posterior cruciate ligament reconstruction using double-double tunnel with tibial anterior and posterior fresh-frozen allograft. Arthroscopy 2006;22(6): 684 e1–5.

[80] Sherman PM, Sanders TG, Morrison WB, et al. MR imaging of the posterior cruciate ligament graft: initial experience in 15 patients with clinical correlation. Radiology 2001;221(1): 191–8.

[81] Buess E, Imhoff AB, Hodler J. Knee evaluation in two systems and magnetic resonance imaging after operative treatment of posterior cruciate ligament injuries. Arch Orthop Trauma Surg 1996; 115(6):307–12.

ELSEVIER
SAUNDERS

RADIOLOGIC
CLINICS
OF NORTH AMERICA

Radiol Clin N Am 45 (2007) 1017–1031

MR Imaging of Synovial Disorders of the Knee: An Update

Matthew A. Frick, MD[a],*, Doris E. Wenger, MD[b], Mark Adkins, MD[c]

- Synovial anatomy and physiology
- MR imaging of the synovium
  Rheumatoid arthritis
  Infectious synovitis
  Pigmented villonodular synovitis

- *Synovial chondromatosis*
  Post-traumatic synovitis
  Synovial tumors
- References

The knee, one of the largest and most complicated joints in the body, is a synovium-lined, diarthrodial articulation consisting of two hinge-type joints between the femoral condyles and the medial and lateral tibial plateaus, and a gliding-type joint between the patella and the trochlear groove of the anterior distal femur. Synovial disorders often affect the knee joint and are a common cause of morbidity. Although the clinician may be able to glean much information about the status of a joint through a combination of physical examination, history, and serologic investigation, direct visualization of the joint at imaging provides invaluable information and often drives important clinical decisions regarding the initiation or modification of therapy.

In the past, radiologists were limited in their ability to provide information about the presence or absence of synovial disease, particularly early in the course of most articular disease processes. Often, radiographs are limited to demonstrating the presence or absence of an effusion and, later,

demonstrating secondary osseous changes. Recent advances in cross-sectional imaging modalities, primarily with MR imaging, but also with CT and ultrasound, have allowed radiologists to provide useful information to referring clinicians about the presence or absence of synovial disorders, often at a time when the initiation of therapy may mitigate significantly the long-term sequelae of a given disorder. White authored an outstanding review of MR imaging of synovial disorders in this series in 1994. This article is a literature-based update regarding the role of MR imaging in the diagnosis and management of synovial disorders of the knee.

Synovial anatomy and physiology

The knee capsule is composed of two layers: an outer fibrous layer and an inner synovial layer, or synovium (Fig. 1). The synovium is a thin membrane that lines the knee capsule and attaches to the margins of the articular surfaces and the periphery of the fibrocartilaginous menisci. Often, a small

This article was originally published in *Magnetic Resonance Imaging Clinics of North America* 15:1, February 2007.
[a] Division of Musculoskeletal Radiology, Department of Radiology, Mayo Clinic and Foundation, 200 First Street SW, Rochester, MN 55905, USA
[b] Division of Musculoskeletal Imaging, Department of Radiology, Mayo Clinic and Foundation, 200 First Street SW, Rochester, MN 55905, USA
[c] Department of Radiology, Mayo Clinic and Foundation, 200 First Street SW, Rochester, MN 55905, USA
* Corresponding author.
E-mail address: frick.matthew@mayo.edu (M.A. Frick).

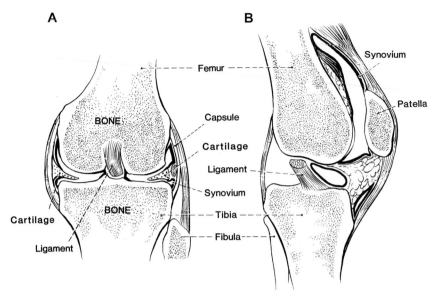

A **B**

Femur

Synovium

Capsule

Patella

BONE

Cartilage

Ligament

Synovium

Cartilage

BONE

Tibia

Ligament

Fibula

Fig. 1. Coronal and sagittal illustrations demonstrate the relationship between the knee capsule, the synovium, and the supporting structures of the knee. Note the intra-articular, but extrasynovial, nature of the cruciate ligaments.

gap exists between the insertion of the synovial membrane/capsule and the nearby articular cartilage, effectively resulting in a "bare area." This area is of significant importance in the pathophysiology and evolution of many arthritides. Anteriorly, the synovial lining extends superiorly, above the patella and deep to the quadriceps femoris, to form the suprapatellar bursa, held in position by a small muscle, the articularis genus, arising from the vastus intermedius. The synovial membrane envelops the anterior and posterior cruciate ligaments so as to exclude them from the "synovial cavity" (ie, these structures are intra-articular but extrasynovial). Posteriorly, the synovial membrane extends caudally on the deep surface of the popliteus tendon, forming the popliteal bursa. An additional bursa, the semimembranosus bursa, lies between the medial head of the gastrocnemius and the medial femoral condyle, and also communicates frequently with the synovial cavity of the joint. These and other less consistent bursae about the knee are discussed in greater detail in this issue by Beaman and colleagues.

On gross inspection, the synovium is a smooth, pink, glistening membrane that contains minute folds, or microvilli, which serve to increase the effective surface area of the joint and allow expansion of the synovial membrane, required for normal joint motion. The inner synovial membrane essentially consists of two layers: a thin layer of lining cells, or intima, and the deeper, more vascular tissues of the subsynovium, consisting of loose connective tissue, fat, fibrous elements, and a rich supply of capillaries and venules. One of the primary functions of the synovium is the secretion of a clear, colorless-to-pale-yellow mucoid substance into the synovial fluid, which facilitates joint lubrication and nutrition. The synovium also plays a critical role in the maintenance of joint integrity by assisting with the removal of debris (ie, cell fragments, particles, and so forth) that may accumulate within the joint during normal wear.

MR imaging of the synovium

The normal synovium is barely perceptible at MR imaging. Visualization of the synovium, therefore, suggests the presence of underlying pathologic change. Although MR imaging is superior to other imaging modalities in its ability to demonstrate abnormal synovium, findings on MR imaging are often nonspecific, owing to the limited number of ways in which the synovium may respond to insult [1]. In general, the pathogenesis of most diseases of the synovium converges on a final common pathway of inflammation, even when the inciting insult is not inflammatory in nature. Following a discussion of the general issues related to MR imaging of synovial disorders about the knee, several distinct disease entities are discussed in detail.

Effusions are a sensitive indicator of joint pathology but, unfortunately, are common in the knee, and may occur in either the presence or absence of proliferative synovitis and thus lack specificity. Synovial thickening or proliferation can be difficult to detect in the presence of a joint effusion with both demonstrating increased signal intensity on fluid-sensitive, or T2-weighted, images (Fig. 2).

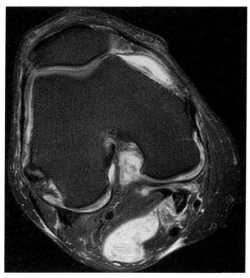

Fig. 2. Axial fat-suppressed T2-weighted MR image from a patient who has rheumatoid arthritis demonstrates the increased signal intensity of both joint effusion/fluid and synovitis.

Electronic review of images on a picture archiving and communications system workstation facilitates the rapid adjustment of window and level settings, which usually allows for confident and easy differentiation of joint fluid and thickened synovium (Fig. 3). Additional morphologic findings may also suggest the presence of an underlying disorder of the synovium. Although somewhat lacking in sensitivity, the presence of scalloping or truncation of the prefemoral fat pad, defects or displacement of Hoffa's fat pad (Fig. 4), and nonvisualization or irregular margins of the quadriceps fat pad have been described as highly specific signs of

synovial proliferation [2]. Administration of intravenous gadolinium–diethylenetriamine pentaacetic acid (DTPA) is also highly accurate in differentiating proliferative synovium from joint effusion (Fig. 5). In the case of rheumatoid arthritis (RA), as discussed later, the rate of synovial enhancement has also been shown to reflect synovial inflammatory activity and may detect subclinical changes [3]. Some investigators have advocated the use of increased doses of gadolinium (0.3 mmol/kg versus 0.1 mmol/kg) as a means of better demonstrating enhancing tissue and reducing the margins of error in the quantification of synovial volume [4,5]. Recent concerns, however, related to the relationship between higher doses of gadolinium and nephrogenic systemic fibrosis, suggest that caution be exercised when contemplating administration of increased doses of intravenous gadolinium.

In addition to being highly sensitive for detecting the presence of joint effusions and synovitis, MR imaging has been shown to be a reliable means of quantifying synovial and effusion volumes. The ability to quantify these synovial processes has important clinical implications regarding the assessment of disease severity and response to therapy [6]. Furthermore, Ostergaard and colleagues [6] have demonstrated that a selected sagittal one-slice volume assessment has high correlation with total joint volumes and is a reliable method of quantifying these parameters. What is not yet certain is whether this measurement may be performed automatically or must be calculated manually.

MR imaging also has been shown to be of value in demonstrating areas of abnormal synovial thickening in patients who have osteoarthritis (OA) and

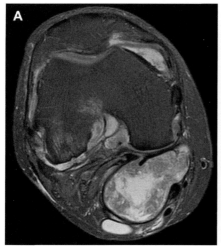 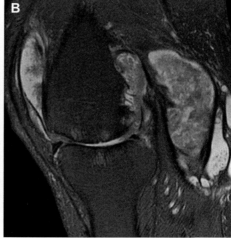

Fig. 3. Axial (*A*) and sagittal (*B*) fat-suppressed T2-weighted MR images from a patient who has known inflammatory arthritis (psoriasis) demonstrate excellent differentiation of joint effusion, which is of high signal intensity, and adjacent synovial thickening and irregularity, which is of intermediate-to-increased signal intensity.

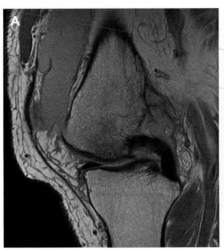
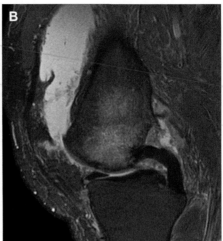

Fig. 4. Sagittal proton density–weighted (*A*) and fat-suppressed T2-weighted (*B*) MR images demonstrate abnormal signal and irregular contour of the infrapatellar (Hoffa's) fat pad in a patient who has known inflammatory arthritis.

is of great value in directing synovial biopsy. In a small study of subjects who had OA of the knee, synovial thickening was seen most commonly in the intercondylar region of the knee, adjacent to the infrapatellar fat pad, or along the posterior margin of the joint [7]. A slightly larger study of 39 subjects who had OA also demonstrated high correlation between areas of synovial thickening at MR imaging and histopathologic findings of active synovitis [8].

Many diseases of the knee, including those arising from, or primarily affecting, the synovium (ie, pigmented villonodular synovitis [PVNS], synovial chondromatosis, hemophilia, synovial tumors, primary OA and rheumatoid, seronegative and infectious arthritis) commonly involve the infrapatellar

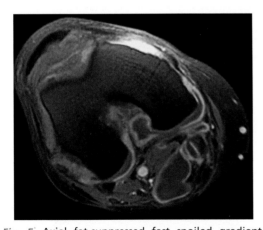

Fig. 5. Axial fat-suppressed fast spoiled gradient-recalled echo MR image of the knee following administration of intravenous gadolinium demonstrates excellent differentiation of enhancing thickened synovium and adjacent joint fluid.

Hoffa's fat pad, either exclusively or as part of total knee involvement, and this region has been shown to be best evaluated with MR imaging [9–11].

Although MR imaging remains the gold standard in the evaluation of synovial disorders of the knee, some investigators have also shown ultrasound to be of correlative accuracy in measurement of synovial thickness [12]. El-Miedany and colleagues [13] found ultrasound to be a simple, inexpensive, and beneficial tool in evaluating the initial stages of juvenile arthritis, but inferior to gadolinium-DTPA–enhanced MR imaging in more advanced stages of the disease and for monitoring response to therapy. The reader is directed to several excellent reports in the literature that describe the use of ultrasound in the diagnosis and management of synovial disorders.

Synovial disorders may be categorized in various ways, including pathogenesis (inflammatory versus noninflammatory), distribution (mono- versus polyarticular), and so forth. Although the synovium is relatively limited in its adaptive responses in the face of insult or injury, it is most useful for discussion purposes to separate disorders of the synovium into inflammatory and noninflammatory categories.

Numerous inflammatory disorders may involve the knee joint, either singularly as a monoarticular process or as part of a systemic, polyarticular process. The most commonly encountered inflammatory arthropathies of the knee include RA, psoriatic arthritis, reactive (Reiter's) arthritis, ankylosing spondylitis, gouty arthritis, and septic arthritis. Because the MR imaging findings in many inflammatory arthropathies are nonspecific and mirror those of RA, the present discussion focuses on the common findings of RA on MR imaging and discusses the merits of MR imaging as the imaging tool of choice for diagnosing and following disease progression. Additional inflammatory arthropathies (ie, seronegative spondyloarthropathies, crystalline deposition disease, and infectious arthropathy) are mentioned briefly. Commonly encountered noninflammatory arthropathies of the knee include OA, posttraumatic synovitis and arthritis, hemorrhagic arthropathies, and several synovial tumor-like entities including PVNS, synovial chondromatosis, and lipoma arborescens.

Rheumatoid arthritis

Rheumatoid arthritis is a common, chronic, and progressive inflammatory disorder characterized by symmetric, bilateral, polyarticular involvement, primarily affecting the synovium. The knees are involved commonly in RA and, in the past, imaging of the knee in rheumatoid patients was limited often to radiographic assessment. Although radiographs may demonstrate both effusion and soft-tissue swelling, their primary usefulness is the demonstration of bony changes (ie, osteopenia,

joint space narrowing, and erosions) that typically occur later in the course of the disease and long after irreversible damage to the joint has occurred. Recent work has shown that instituting therapy with disease-modifying antirheumatic drugs early in the course of the disease, often as early as the first several months, has a significant effect on long-term prognosis and disease progression. Although much of the work to date evaluating the role of MR imaging in early detection and quantification of RA has centered on imaging of the hands and wrists, the findings of these studies generally are referable to the knee. MR imaging has been shown to be clearly superior to conventional radiographs for the demonstration of early or occult changes of RA, namely synovitis and effusion (Fig. 6) [14,15]. The presence of synovitis is considered a strong predictor of future erosive changes [16]. Similarly, MR imaging has been found to be superior in the detection of early findings of juvenile idiopathic arthritis [17]. In a series of 86 subjects who had RA of the knee, Takeuchi and colleagues [18] devised a 10-item quantitative analysis based on MR imaging findings that classified the severity of symptoms

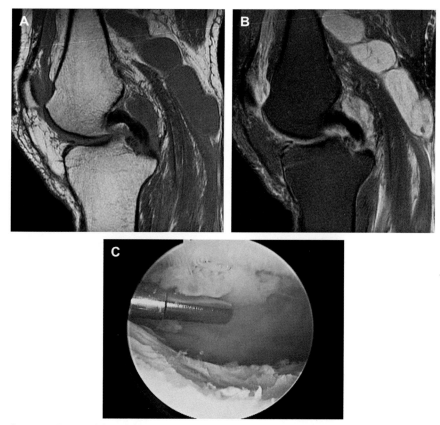

Fig. 6. Sagittal proton density (*A*) and fat-suppressed T2-weighted (*B*) MR images of the knee from a patient who has RA demonstrate marked synovial thickening and irregularity, joint effusion, and evidence of synovitis within a large popliteal cyst. Arthroscopic image (*C*) demonstrates thickened, irregular synovium.

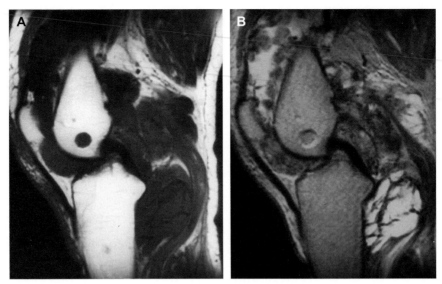

Fig. 7. Sagittal T1-weighted (*A*) and T2-weighted (*B*) MR images of the knee demonstrate characteristic features of PVNS with massive distention of the joint by nodular, low T1 and T2 signal intensity, intra-articular masses, and joint effusion. The circular focus of low signal intensity within the distal femur was shown on additional images to represent a small erosion.

into four grades (score 0 to 3). In their study, synovial proliferation was scored highly in the early stages of the disease, suggesting that it was the initial finding of RA. This scale was shown further to have usefulness for following the progression of disease and response to therapy.

As discussed previously, MR imaging has become a central tool in the evaluation of RA because of its superior soft-tissue contrast, its ability to detect and quantify synovial thickening/volume, and the fact that this measurement correlates highly with synovial inflammatory activity [19]. MR imaging, owing to its superior contrast, is capable of demonstrating periarticular soft-tissue swelling, bone marrow changes, and abnormalities of the adjacent tendons and ligaments. MR imaging has also been shown to be highly accurate in documenting the presence of entheseal abnormalities about the knee, which are encountered commonly in patients who have spondyloarthropathy but not RA, a differentiation which has important diagnostic, treatment, and prognostic implications [20]. Acute synovial rupture, a rare complication of RA, has also been shown to be seen well on MR imaging [21].

Although every MR imaging examination should be tailored to answer the clinical question at hand, routine MR imaging sequences have been shown to be highly accurate in identifying the presence and extent of synovial abnormalities. Bredella and colleagues [22] devised a grading scheme for synovial thickening (grade 0 = normal, grade 1 = thin line of increased signal intensity, and grade 2 = increased signal intensity with frond-like or hair-like

projections and a granular appearance of the joint fluid) that showed MR to be highly sensitive and specific when compared with arthroscopy. In their experience, proton density and T2-weighted fast-spin echo or spin-echo sequences with fat saturation in the axial and sagittal planes were most useful.

Although fat-suppressed T1-weighted 3D gradient-echo images offer sufficient differentiation of cartilage and joint fluid in patients who have RA of the knees, it is recognized generally that

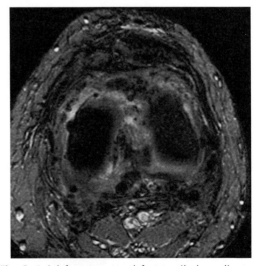

Fig. 8. Axial fat-suppressed fast spoiled gradient-recalled echo MR image of the knee demonstrates characteristic "blooming" artifact seen in PVNS, which occurs on gradient-echo sequences because of the T2* effect of paramagnetic hemosiderin.

gadolinium-DTPA–enhanced MR images offer superior differentiation of enlarged or hyperplastic synovium from adjacent joint fluid [17,23]. A potential pitfall is that MR imaging also detects synovial enhancement in "normal" volunteers or control subjects and, aside from demonstrable thickening and irregularity, no discrete criteria differentiate this normal enhancement from the presumed abnormal enhancement that occurs in RA and other inflammatory arthropathies [24].

Much research interest has centered around the assessment of dynamic gadolinium enhancement of the synovium in patients who have RA [25–28]. The rate of early enhancement (30 to 60 seconds following injection) has been shown to correlate highly with microscopic evidence of active inflammation (vessel proliferation and mononuclear leukocyte infiltration) and has high predictive value in distinguishing knees without and with synovial inflammation [26]. The rate of synovial

enhancement on gadolinium-DTPA–enhanced MR imaging has also been shown to correlate with blood vessel density and fractional area, which may prove valuable in evaluating drugs that influence angiogenesis, an area of active pharmaceutic research [29]. The distinction between synovium and joint fluid is most reliable in the first 10 minutes following injection of gadolinium contrast because the gadolinium diffuses into the joint, thereby obscuring the border between synovium and effusion [28].

Several investigators have shown MR imaging to be highly reliable and accurate when used to follow disease progression and monitor response to therapy, and also to detect recurrence of disease following synovectomy [16,30]. In addition to disease-modifying antirheumatic drugs, intra-articular steroid injections are a commonly used treatment in RA, and MR imaging has been shown to assess the effect of treatment quantitatively [31]. The

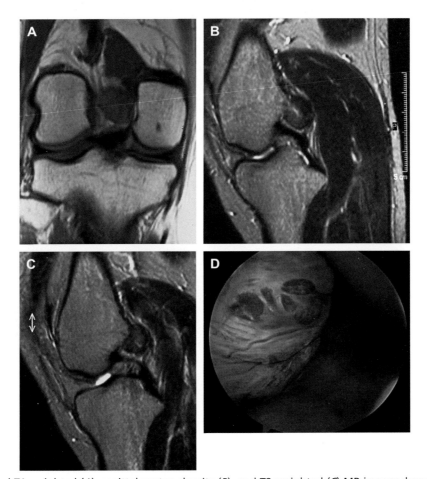

Fig. 9. Coronal T1-weighted (*A*), sagittal proton density (*B*), and T2-weighted (*C*) MR images demonstrate focal nodular PVNS. The focal mass in the posterior intercondylar region demonstrates characteristic decreased signal intensity on all pulse sequences. Corresponding arthroscopic image (*D*) demonstrates hemosiderin pigment deposition responsible for the characteristic MR imaging appearance.

effects of radiosynovectomy, performed by way of the intra-articular injection of a radiopharmaceutic agent to ameliorate the synovial inflammatory process, may also be evaluated with gadolinium-DTPA–enhanced MR imaging [32,33].

Infectious synovitis

Infectious arthritis of the knee may occur because of bacterial, viral, fungal, or other microbial organisms. This topic is addressed in depth by Bancroft and colleagues elsewhere in this issue and is not discussed further here other than to reiterate the critical importance of early recognition and treatment of infectious arthritis and the importance of maintaining a high level of suspicion and a readiness to perform, or recommend, joint aspiration, because the MR findings, consisting of synovial thickening, joint fluid, and possible septations or debris, are relatively nonspecific. Aspiration of joint fluid should not be delayed to obtain an MR image because this may result in an unnecessary delay in treatment.

Pigmented villonodular synovitis

The term pigmented villonodular synovitis was used first by Jaffe in 1941 to describe an uncommon, benign process characterized histologically by hyperplastic synovial proliferation either within joints, along tendon sheaths and periarticular fascial planes, or within bursae. When occurring outside the joint, the disorder is referred to as giant cell tumor of the tendon sheath.

The exact cause of PVNS is unclear. Some investigators believe that PVNS represents a chronic inflammatory response, whereas others have suggested that PVNS represents a benign neoplasm of fibrohistiocytic origin [34]. Localized (nodular) and diffuse forms of the disease may occur in the knee, with the latter being the predominant form. As many as 80% of all cases of the diffuse form of PVNS occur in the knee [35]. The disorder most commonly presents between the second and fourth decades of life, with no sex predilection, manifesting as a painful knee and often with recurrent sanguineous effusions.

Histologic evaluation demonstrates hypertrophied synovium containing, in addition to multinucleated giant cells and histiocytes, a significant amount of both intra- and extracellular hemosiderin pigment, which accounts for the characteristic MR imaging appearance of this disorder. The paramagnetic effects of hemosiderin result in areas of low signal intensity on both T1 and T2-weighted images (Fig. 7) [36,37]. Although this finding is highly suggestive of PVNS, the most characteristic finding is prominent "blooming" artifact in these same regions on gradient-echo images (Fig. 8),

which occurs because of the signal decay (T2*-effect) of hemosiderin-laden thickened synovium and masses [38]. The MR imaging features of PVNS include nodular low T1 and T2 signal intensity masses bathed in surrounding high T2 signal intensity joint fluid, with or without cystic changes and erosions of the adjacent joint surfaces [39]. Common sites of involvement include the suprapatellar bursa, the infrapatellar fat pad, and posterior to the cruciate ligaments. Often, PVNS of the hip and other less capacious joints is characterized by prominent osseous changes; however, PVNS of the knee is associated commonly with minimal joint or bone destruction [37]. Postgadolinium images may demonstrate variable degrees of enhancement, particularly in nodules containing minimal hemosiderin 35, and, although rarely a diagnostic dilemma, PVNS has been shown to demonstrate a slower enhancement rate compared with those seen in the inflammatory arthropathies, namely RA [40]. However, in a large series of 44 subjects, Barile and colleagues [41] found that gadolinium-enhanced images provided no additional diagnostic MR information.

Localized, or focal, nodular PVNS of the knee is uncommon, and may present as a discrete, pedunculated mass protruding into the articular cavity that clinically may result in mechanical symptoms such as locking [42]. The knee is the most commonly affected joint in localized, or focal, nodular forms of PVNS (Fig. 9) and, in contrast to the diffuse form, complete recovery or cure is achieved relatively easily, with only rare reports of recurrence [43].

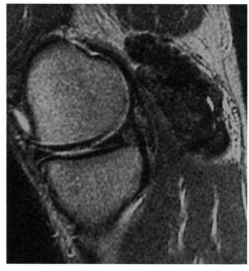

Fig. 10. Sagittal T2-weighted MR image of the knee demonstrates changes of PVNS within a popliteal cyst, a location which would not be visualized arthroscopically.

MR imaging provides a highly accurate map of joint involvement, which is of central importance for preoperative planning and postoperative follow-up [44,45]. MR imaging is helpful for defining the total extent of disease, specifically in recesses or areas that may be missed by arthroscopy alone (for example, along the popliteus tendon, or within a popliteal cyst) (Fig. 10). Arthroscopic synovectomy has been shown to be an appropriate treatment for PVNS of the knee. In a series of 19 subjects (4 with localized disease and 15 with diffuse involvement), De Ponti and colleagues [46] found that arthroscopic local excision was curative in the all subjects who had focal disease, and that extended synovectomy (versus partial synovectomy) led to better clinical results and lower

recurrence rates with no significant complications encountered. However, recurrence rates remain high in cases of diffuse PVNS.

Synovial chondromatosis

Synovial chondromatosis is a monoarticular process characterized histologically by metaplasia of the synovium leading to the generation of lobulated, pedunculated, cartilaginous foci, which often shed into the joint and which may or may not ossify/calcify (osteochondromatosis). The knees, and other large joints such as the hips and elbows, are involved most commonly.

The histologic nature of the bodies determines their MR imaging appearance. Cartilaginous foci, which are often occult radiographically,

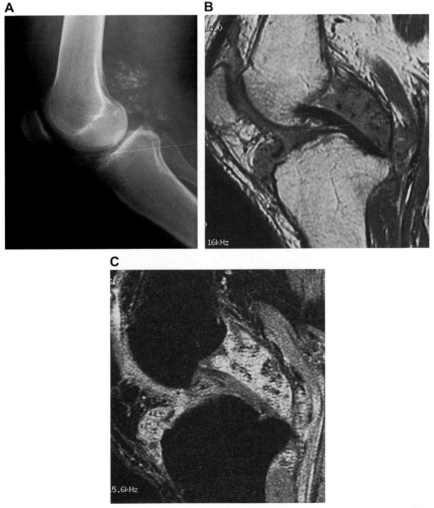

Fig. 11. Lateral radiograph (*A*) of the knee demonstrates multiple tiny osteocartilaginous bodies of relatively uniform size within the posterior aspect of the knee joint. Sagittal T1-weighted (*B*) and fat-suppressed T2-weighted (*C*) MR images of the knee from a patient who has surgically proven synovial osteochondromatosis demonstrate low signal intensity bodies throughout the knee joint, with associated synovial thickening and joint effusion.

demonstrate intermediate T1 and T2 signal intensity. Noncalcified bodies may be difficult to differentiate from high signal intensity joint fluid on fluid-sensitive sequences. Calcified foci tend to demonstrate low signal intensity on both T1- and T2-weighted sequences. Lesions that are osseous or osteocartilaginous tend to mirror bone marrow on MR imaging, with hyperintense signal intensity on non–fat-suppressed images and intermediate to low T2 signal intensity, depending on the presence or absence of fat-saturated sequences (Fig. 11). In a few cases, synovial chondromatosis may be occult radiographically with no detectable calcification, and patients may present to MR imaging with nonspecific symptoms [47]. In this setting, the radiologist may be the first to suggest the diagnosis.

Synovial chondromatosis is treated most commonly with either open or arthroscopic synovectomy. Although usually this is curative, recurrent synovial chondromatosis may occur and, in a few case reports, may be highly refractory [48]. Although rare, malignant degeneration of synovial chondromatosis may occur, often with no distinctive MR imaging features that allow differentiation of these lesions from those of benign primary synovial chondromatosis [49].

Post-traumatic synovitis

In response to acute insult or injury, the vasculature of the subsynovium vasodilates and becomes edematous, resulting in intermediate T1 and increased T2 signal intensity that makes the

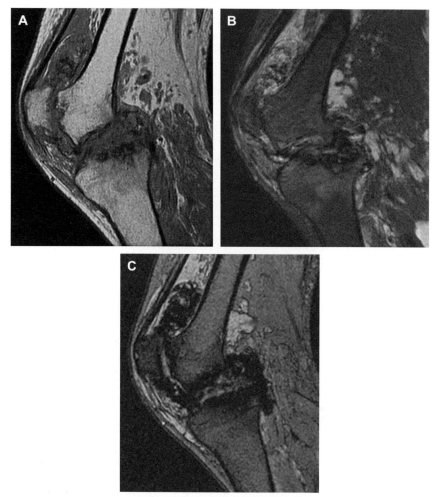

Fig. 12. Sagittal T1-weighted (*A*) and T2-weighted (*B*) MR images of the knee from a patient who has Klippel-Trenaunay syndrome with a known history of multiple knee hemarthroses demonstrate marked destructive changes in the knee, with a large joint effusion containing extensive areas of decreased signal intensity. These foci of low signal intensity demonstrate significant "blooming" artifact on the corresponding sagittal gradient-recalled echo image (*C*). Typical changes of Klippel-Trenaunay syndrome with vascular malformations are also present in the adjacent soft tissues.

differentiation of synovium from effusion difficult or impossible. With continued synovial inflammation, the irregularly thickened synovium becomes more prominent and easier to differentiate from adjacent fluid [50]. Continued or chronic injury leads to adhesions and fibrosis. Occasionally, large inflammatory masses may develop along with evidence of joint destruction.

Commonly, patients who have hemophilia and other bleeding diatheses are beset by recurrent hemorrhagic effusions, often in the knee and other large joints, which culminate ultimately in arthropathy with almost universal involvement of the synovium. As a result of repeated hemarthrosis, the knee joint has a considerable deposition of hemosiderin pigment, predominantly within the synovium, resulting in characteristic decreased T1 and T2 signal

intensity and the expected "blooming" artifact on gradient-echo images (Fig. 12). MR imaging with gradient-echo and contrast-enhanced sequences has been shown to be superior to clinical examination for the detection of intra-articular blood products and provides additional useful clinical information regarding the early stages of synovial and cartilage alteration, which may assist therapy planning [51].

The findings of chronic hemophilic arthropathy may mimic those of PVNS, as discussed earlier. Differentiating factors in favor of hemophilic arthropathy include lack of prominent nodularity, more pronounced cartilage, and subchondral bone injury, and, in some instances, widening of the intercondylar notch. Additionally, although many patients presenting with findings of PVNS on MR

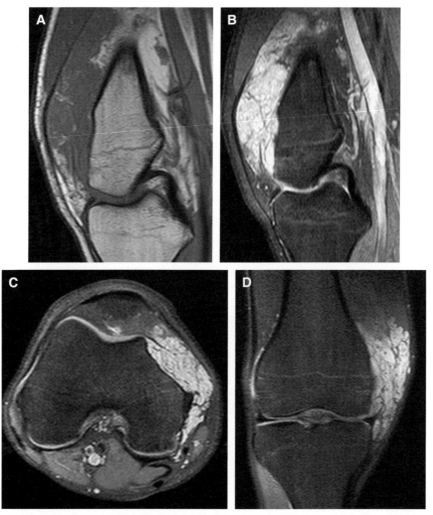

Fig. 13. Sagittal T1-weighted (*A*) and fat-suppressed T2-weighted (*B*) MR images of the knee demonstrate a large intra-articular mass that has a lobulated morphology and contains linear foci of fat. The fat-suppressed axial (*C*) and coronal (*D*) T2-weighted images demonstrate the intra- and juxta-articular nature of this mass. This lesion was resected surgically and shown to represent a hemangioma.

imaging often have no pre-imaging diagnosis, patients who have hemophilic arthropathy typically have a documented history of the disorder.

As with other disorders discussed in this article, in addition to diagnosing the presence and extent of hemophilic changes, MR imaging plays a central role in the longitudinal assessment of response to therapy and disease progression. Two MR imaging scoring systems have been devised for the assessment of hemophilic arthropathy, and preliminary studies have shown high intra- and interobserver reliability [52]. Although MR imaging may provide useful diagnostic information following radiosynoviorthesis, pretreatment scans have failed to show any meaningful predictions regarding response to therapy [53].

Synovial tumors

Hemangiomas, or vascular malformations, of the synovium are rare and may represent a difficult problem in diagnosis and treatment. Lesions may present in one of two forms, either as a synovial hemangioma or as an arteriovenous malformation referred to as a hemangiohamartoma, both of which involve the synovium and often present with a long history of joint pain and nontraumatic episodes of hemarthrosis [54].

In a small series of five subjects who had surgically proven synovial hemangiomas, a diagnostic delay averaging 8 years had occurred in four of the cases because radiographs, and even CT and arteriography, are often nondiagnostic. In this series, synovial hemangiomas demonstrated increased T2 signal intensity without significant mass effect. Additional features were fibrofatty septa and muscular or fatty invasion [55]. A larger series of eight subjects showed MR imaging to be superior to other imaging modalities, and in all cases demonstrated

an intra- or juxta-articular mass of intermediate signal intensity on T1-weighted images and of high signal intensity on T2-weighted images, with low-signal channels or septa within the lesions (Fig. 13) [56]. Administration of contrast material often may demonstrate avid, rather homogeneous enhancement, which may allow differentiation from cystic synovial hyperplasia. The latter may be confused with cavernous synovial hemangiomas, but tend to demonstrate less intense, peripheral enhancement [57]. Treatment is complete, open synovectomy.

Lipoma arborescens (diffuse articular lipomatosis) is a rare, benign villous lipomatous proliferation of the synovium of unknown cause that occurs most commonly in the knee. Antecedent trauma or chronic inflammatory conditions have been suggested as predisposing factors, but the disorder may also occur in individuals with no such history. Although typically monoarticular, case reports of bilateral lipoma arborescens of the knee have been reported [58,59]. Additionally, at least three cases have been reported of simultaneous polyarticular involvement in patients, which may mimic an inflammatory arthropathy [60]. Clinically, the most common presentation is a slowly enlarging, swollen joint, often with evidence of an effusion. At MR imaging, the villous lipomatous proliferation demonstrates signal characteristics similar to fat on both T1- and T2-weighted sequences, and may also demonstrate subsynovial fat deposition in approximately one third of cases (Fig. 14) [61]. Although most often diffuse in nature and centered most commonly in the suprapatellar recess, focal forms of lipoma arborescens may occur in as many as 20% of cases [62]. One series of 13 subjects described three distinct morphologic patterns on MR imaging; multiple villous

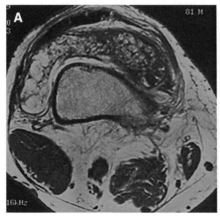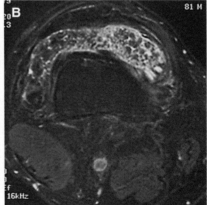

Fig. 14. Axial T1-weighted (*A*) and fat-suppressed T2-weighted (*B*) MR images of the knee demonstrate nodular frond-like masses within the suprapatellar recess that have the signal intensity of fat, with surrounding joint fluid consistent with lipoma arborescens.

lipomatous synovial proliferations (n = 6), isolated, frond-like, fat subsynovial mass (n = 2), and a mixed pattern (n = 5) [63]. Lipoma arborescens is also associated almost invariably with additional intra-articular pathology, most commonly joint effusions and changes of degenerative arthritis [62].

In summary, MR imaging, owing to its superior soft-tissue contrast, is the imaging modality of choice for demonstrating and quantifying pathologic changes of the synovium and provides invaluable information to the clinician regarding the need to either initiate or modify therapy in those patients suffering from diseases of, or affecting, the synovium.

References

[1] Suh JS, Griffiths HJ, Galloway HR, et al. Radiologic case study. MRI in the diagnosis of synovial disease. Orthopedics 1992;15(6):774, 778–81.

[2] Schweitzer ME, Falk A, Pathria M, et al. MR imaging of the knee: can changes in the intracapsular fat pads be used as a sign of synovial proliferation in the presence of an effusion? AJR Am J Roentgenol 1993;160(4):823–6.

[3] Ostergaard M, Stoltenberg M, Henriksen O, et al. Quantitative assessment of synovial inflammation by dynamic gadolinium-enhanced magnetic resonance imaging. A study of the effect of intra-articular methylprednisolone on the rate of early synovial enhancement. Br J Rheumatol 1996; 35(1):50–9.

[4] Oliver C, Speake S, Watt I, et al. Advantages of an increased dose of MRI contrast agent for enhancing inflammatory synovium. Clin Radiol 1996; 51(7):487–93.

[5] Oliver C, Watt I. Intravenous MRI contrast enhancement of inflammatory synovium: a dose study. Br J Rheumatol 1996;35(Suppl 3):31–5.

[6] Ostergaard M, Gideon P, Henriksen O, et al. Synovial volume–a marker of disease severity in rheumatoid arthritis? Quantification by MRI. Scand J Rheumatol 1994;23(4):197–202.

[7] Fernandez-Madrid F, Karvonen RL, Teitge RA, et al. Synovial thickening detected by MR imaging in osteoarthritis of the knee confirmed by biopsy as synovitis. Magn Reson Imaging 1995; 13(2):177–83.

[8] Loeuille D, Chary-Valckenaere I, Champigneulle J, et al. Macroscopic and microscopic features of synovial membrane inflammation in the osteoarthritic knee: correlating magnetic resonance imaging findings with disease severity. Arthritis Rheum 2005;52(11):3492–501.

[9] Jacobson JA, Lenchik L, Ruhoy MK, et al. MR imaging of the infrapatellar fat pad of Hoffa. Radiographics 1997;17(3):675–91.

[10] Saddik D, McNally EG, Richardson M. MRI of Hoffa's fat pad. Skeletal Radiol 2004;33(8): 433–44.

[11] Ozkur A, Adaletli I, Sirikci A, et al. Hoffa's recess in the infrapatellar fat pad of the knee on MR imaging. Surg Radiol Anat 2005;27(1):61–3.

[12] Ostergaard M, Court-Payen M, Gideon P, et al. Ultrasonography in arthritis of the knee. A comparison with MR imaging. Acta Radiol 1995; 36(1):19–26.

[13] El-Miedany YM, Housny IH, Mansour HM, et al. Ultrasound versus MRI in the evaluation of juvenile idiopathic arthritis of the knee. Joint Bone Spine 2001;68(3):222–30.

[14] Forslind K, Larsson EM, Johansson A, et al. Detection of joint pathology by magnetic resonance imaging in patients with early rheumatoid arthritis. Br J Rheumatol 1997;36(6):683–8.

[15] Forslind K, Larsson EM, Eberhardt K, et al. Magnetic resonance imaging of the knee: a tool for prediction of joint damage in early rheumatoid arthritis? Scand J Rheumatol 2004;33(3): 154–61.

[16] Ostergaard M, Hansen M, Stoltenberg M, et al. Magnetic resonance imaging-determined synovial membrane volume as a marker of disease activity and a predictor of progressive joint destruction in the wrists of patients with rheumatoid arthritis. Arthritis Rheum 1999;42(5): 918–29.

[17] Johnson K, Wittkop B, Haigh F, et al. The early magnetic resonance imaging features of the knee in juvenile idiopathic arthritis. Clin Radiol 2002;57(6):466–71.

[18] Takeuchi K, Inoue H, Yokoyama Y, et al. Evaluation of rheumatoid arthritis using a scoring system devised from magnetic resonance imaging of rheumatoid knees. Acta Med Okayama 1998;52(4):211–24.

[19] Ostergaard M, Stoltenberg M, Lovgreen-Nielsen P, et al. Magnetic resonance imaging-determined synovial membrane and joint effusion volumes in rheumatoid arthritis and osteoarthritis: comparison with the macroscopic and microscopic appearance of the synovium. Arthritis Rheum 1997;40(10):1856–67.

[20] McGonagle D, Gibbon W, O'Connor P, et al. Characteristic magnetic resonance imaging entheseal changes of knee synovitis in spondyloarthropathy. Arthritis Rheum 1998;41(4): 694–700.

[21] Yamamoto T, Marui T, Akisue T, et al. Acute synovial rupture of the rheumatoid knee presenting as a pretibial mass: MRI appearance. J Rheumatol 2003;30(5):1097–9.

[22] Bredella MA, Tirman PF, Wischer TK, et al. Reactive synovitis of the knee joint: MR imaging appearance with arthroscopic correlation. Skeletal Radiol 2000;29(10):577–82.

[23] Rand T, Imhof H, Czerny C, et al. Discrimination between fluid, synovium, and cartilage in patients with rheumatoid arthritis: contrast enhanced spin echo versus non-contrast-enhanced fat-suppressed gradient echo MR imaging. Clin Radiol 1999;54(2):107–10.

[24] Ejbjerg B, Narvestad E, Rostrup E, et al. Magnetic resonance imaging of wrist and finger joints in healthy subjects occasionally shows changes resembling erosions and synovitis as seen in rheumatoid arthritis. Arthritis Rheum 2004;50(4): 1097–106.

[25] Ostergaard M, Lorenzen I, Henriksen O. Dynamic gadolinium-enhanced MR imaging in active and inactive immunoinflammatory gonarthritis. Acta Radiol 1994;35(3):275–81.

[26] Ostergaard M, Stoltenberg M, Lovgreen-Nielsen P, et al. Quantification of synovitis by MRI: correlation between dynamic and static gadolinium-enhanced magnetic resonance imaging and microscopic and macroscopic signs of synovial inflammation. Magn Reson Imaging 1998;16(7):743–54.

[27] Doria AS, Noseworthy M, Oakden W, et al. Dynamic contrast-enhanced MRI quantification of synovium microcirculation in experimental arthritis. 10.2214/AJR.04.1138. AJR Am J Roentgenol 2006;186(4):1165–71.

[28] Ostergaard M, Klarlund M. Importance of timing of post-contrast MRI in rheumatoid arthritis: what happens during the first 60 minutes after IV gadolinium-DTPA? Ann Rheum Dis 2001; 60(11):1050–4.

[29] Gaffney K, Cookson J, Blades S, et al. Quantitative assessment of the rheumatoid synovial microvascular bed by gadolinium-DTPA enhanced magnetic resonance imaging. Ann Rheum Dis 1998;57(3):152–7.

[30] Ostergaard M, Ejbjerg B, Stoltenberg M, et al. Quantitative magnetic resonance imaging as marker of synovial membrane regeneration and recurrence of synovitis after arthroscopic knee joint synovectomy: a one year follow up study. Ann Rheum Dis 2001;60(3):233–6.

[31] Creamer P, Keen M, Zananiri F, et al. Quantitative magnetic resonance imaging of the knee: a method of measuring response to intra-articular treatments. Ann Rheum Dis 1997;56(6): 378–81.

[32] Alonso-Ruiz A, Perez-Ruiz F, Calabozo M, et al. Efficacy of radiosynovectomy of the knee in rheumatoid arthritis: evaluation with magnetic resonance imaging. Clin Rheumatol 1998; 17(4):277–81.

[33] Lee SH, Suh JS, Kim HS, et al. MR evaluation of radiation synovectomy of the knee by means of intra-articular injection of holmium-166-chitosan complex in patients with rheumatoid arthritis: results at 4-month follow-up. Korean J Radiol 2003;4(3):170–8.

[34] Goldman AB, DiCarlo EF. Pigmented villonodular synovitis. Diagnosis and differential diagnosis. Radiol Clin North Am 1988;26(6): 1327–47.

[35] Dorwart RH, Genant HK, Johnston WH, et al. Pigmented villonodular synovitis of synovial joints: clinical, pathologic, and radiologic features. AJR Am J Roentgenol 1984;143(4):877–85.

[36] Araki Y, Tanaka H, Yamamoto H, et al. MR imaging of pigmented villonodular synovitis of the knee. Radiat Med 1994;12(1):11–5.

[37] Cheng XG, You YH, Liu W, et al. MRI features of pigmented villonodular synovitis (PVNS). Clin Rheumatol 2004;23(1):31–4.

[38] Eckhardt BP, Hernandez RJ. Pigmented villonodular synovitis: MR imaging in pediatric patients. Pediatr Radiol 2004;34(12):943–7.

[39] Hughes TH, Sartoris DJ, Schweitzer ME, et al. Pigmented villonodular synovitis: MRI characteristics. Skeletal Radiol 1995;24(1):7–12.

[40] Dale K, Smith HJ, Paus AC, et al. Dynamic MR-imaging in the diagnosis of pigmented villonodular synovitis of the knee. Scand J Rheumatol 2000;29(5):336–9.

[41] Barile A, Sabatini M, Iannessi F, et al. Pigmented villonodular synovitis (PVNS) of the knee joint: magnetic resonance imaging (MRI) using standard and dynamic paramagnetic contrast media. Report of 52 cases surgically and histologically controlled. Radiol Med (Torino) 2004;107(4): 356–66.

[42] Delcogliano A, Galli M, Menghi A, et al. Localized pigmented villonodular synovitis of the knee: report of two cases of fat pad involvement. Arthroscopy 1998;14(5):527–31.

[43] Asik M, Erlap L, Altinel L, et al. Localized pigmented villonodular synovitis of the knee. Arthroscopy 2001;17(6):E23.

[44] Steinbach LS, Neumann CH, Stoller DW, et al. MRI of the knee in diffuse pigmented villonodular synovitis. Clin Imaging 1989;13(4):305–16.

[45] Iovane A, Midiri M, Bartolotta TV, et al. Pigmented villonodular synovitis of the foot: MR findings. Radiol Med (Torino) 2003;106(1–2): 66–73.

[46] De Ponti A, Sansone V, Malchere M. Result of arthroscopic treatment of pigmented villonodular synovitis of the knee. Arthroscopy 2003;19(6): 602–7.

[47] Lin RC, Lue KH, Lin ZI, et al. Primary synovial chondromatosis mimicking medial meniscal tear in a young man. Arthroscopy 2006;22(7): 803, 801–3.

[48] Church JS, Breidahl WH, Janes GC. Recurrent synovial chondromatosis of the knee after radical synovectomy and arthrodesis. J Bone Joint Surg Br 2006;88(5):673–5.

[49] Wittkop B, Davies AM, Mangham DC. Primary synovial chondromatosis and synovial chondrosarcoma: a pictorial review. Eur Radiol 2002; 12(8):2112–9.

[50] White EM. Magnetic resonance imaging in synovial disorders and arthropathy of the knee. Magn Reson Imaging Clin N Am 1994;2(3):451–61.

[51] Rand T, Trattnig S, Male C, et al. Magnetic resonance imaging in hemophilic children: value of gradient echo and contrast-enhanced imaging. Magn Reson Imaging 1999;17(2):199–205.

[52] Doria AS, Lundin B, Kilcoyne RF, et al. Reliability of progressive and additive MRI scoring systems

for evaluation of haemophilic arthropathy in children: expert MRI Working Group of the International Prophylaxis Study Group. Haemophilia 2005;11(3):245–53.

[53] Nuss R, Kilcoyne RF, Geraghty S, et al. MRI findings in haemophilic joints treated with radiosynoviorthesis with development of an MRI scale of joint damage. Haemophilia 2000;6(3):162–9.

[54] Yercan HS, Okcu G, Erkan S. Synovial hemangiohamartomas of the knee joint. Arch Orthop Trauma Surg Apr 12, 2006.

[55] Cotten A, Flipo RM, Herbaux B, et al. Synovial haemangioma of the knee: a frequently misdiagnosed lesion. Skeletal Radiol 1995;24(4): 257–61.

[56] Greenspan A, Azouz EM, Matthews J 2nd, et al. Synovial hemangioma: imaging features in eight histologically proven cases, review of the literature, and differential diagnosis. Skeletal Radiol 1995;24(8):583–90.

[57] De Filippo M, Rovani C, Sudberry JJ, et al. Magnetic resonance imaging comparison of intra-articular cavernous synovial hemangioma and cystic synovial hyperplasia of the knee. Acta Radiol 2006;47(6):581–4.

[58] Cil A, Atay OA, Aydingoz U, et al. Bilateral lipoma arborescens of the knee in a child: a case report. Knee Surg Sports Traumatol Arthrosc 2005;13(6):463–7.

[59] Davies AP, Blewitt N. Lipoma arborescens of the knee. Knee 2005;12(5):394–6.

[60] Bejia I, Younes M, Moussa A, et al. Lipoma arborescens affecting multiple joints. Skeletal Radiol 2005;34(9):536–8.

[61] Ryu KN, Jaovisidha S, Schweitzer M, et al. MR imaging of lipoma arborescens of the knee joint. AJR Am J Roentgenol 1996;167(5):1229–32.

[62] Vilanova JC, Barcelo J, Villalon M, et al. MR imaging of lipoma arborescens and the associated lesions. Skeletal Radiol 2003;32(9):504–9.

[63] Soler T, Rodriguez E, Bargiela A, et al. Lipoma arborescens of the knee: MR characteristics in 13 joints. J Comput Assist Tomogr 1998;22(4): 605–9.

RADIOLOGIC
CLINICS
OF NORTH AMERICA

Radiol Clin N Am 45 (2007) 1033–1053

MR Imaging of the Meniscus: Review, Current Trends, and Clinical Implications

Michael G. Fox, MD

The use of MR imaging to diagnose meniscal pathology is extremely common. The sensitivity and specificity for MR imaging in diagnosing meniscal tears in patients without prior surgery varies, depending on the study; however, the consensus is that MR imaging is accurate in this patient population. Because the meniscus plays an important role in the structure and function of the knee, and the absence of a normal meniscus can lead to accelerated and irreversible degenerative changes [1,2], meniscal repair, and even transplantation, have become more common. Evaluation of the postoperative knee is more complicated, and the best imaging technique for these patients is often debated. A through knowledge of meniscal anatomy, meniscal variants, meniscal tears, and the expected postoperative appearance of repaired or partially resected menisci is required, to provide the referring clinician with useful information for patient management.

Anatomy

The menisci are wedge-shaped, semilunar (C-shaped), fibrocartilage structures composed of thick collagen fibers primarily arranged circumferentially, with radial fibers extending from the capsule, between the circumferential fibers. The superior

This article was originally published in *Magnetic Resonance Imaging Clinics of North America* 15:1, February 2007.
Division of Musculoskeletal Radiology, Department of Radiology, University of Virginia, Box 800170, Charlottesville, VA 22908, USA
E-mail address: mf3kx@hscmail.mcc.virginia.edu

doi:10.1016/j.rcl.2007.08.009

surface of the meniscus is concave and the inferior surface is flat, allowing for maximal congruency between the femur and tibia. With weight bearing, the curved femoral condylar surfaces radially displace the menisci, creating circumferential hoop stresses. The circumferential arrangement of the type I collagen fibers provides the meniscus with tensile strength [2]. The menisci transmit more than 50% of body weight in extension, and even more in flexion [3]. These properties allow the meniscus to perform many functions, including the distribution of stresses over the articular cartilage, the absorption of shocks during axial loading, the stabilization of the joint in both flexion and extension, and joint lubrication; they also make a minor contribution toward secondary stabilization of the knee after cruciate ligament injuries [1,2].

The menisci cover 50% of the medial and 70% of the lateral surface of the tibial plateau [1]. Typically, the medial meniscus is larger, has a wider posterior horn, and is more "open" toward the intercondylar notch, with the lateral meniscus typically smaller and more "closed" toward the notch. In adults, the vascularized area, commonly known as the "red zone," involves the outer 10% to 30% of the meniscus [1,4]. Each meniscus is divided arbitrarily into an anterior horn, a body, and a posterior horn. Usually, the anterior horn of the medial meniscus is attached to the tibial plateau anterior to the anterior cruciate ligament (ACL) [1]. The anterior horn of the lateral meniscus has fibers of the ACL that extend into it at the anterior root attachment where it attaches to the tibial plateau. The transverse or anterior intermeniscal ligament, which is noted in 44% to 58% of patients on MR, has variable attachments; however, 58% of the time it runs between the anterior horn of the medial meniscus and the anterior margin of the lateral meniscus, connecting the two anterior horns [5]. The posterior horn of the lateral meniscus attaches to the posterior tibia, and usually has attachments to the medial femoral condyle and the popliteus by way of the meniscofemoral ligaments and the popliteomeniscal fascicles, respectively. The posterior horn of the medial meniscus attaches to the tibial plateau immediately anterior to the posterior cruciate ligament (PCL) [1].

The meniscofemoral ligaments extend from the posterior horn lateral meniscus usually to the lateral aspect of the posterior medial femoral condyle, but occasionally to the PCL. The incidence of at least one meniscofemoral ligament identified on MR ranges from 66% to 93%, with both identified in anatomic studies more than 30% of the time [6,7]. Typically, when both are present, one is notably thicker. They have properties similar to the posterior bundle of the PCL and may supplement the PCL, providing secondary restraint. The ligament of Humphrey is anterior and the ligament of Wrisberg is posterior to the PCL (Fig. 1). The meniscofemoral ligaments oppose the posterior movement of the posterior horn of the lateral meniscus and "pull" the posterior horn of the lateral meniscus anteriorly and medially [6]. The popliteomeniscal fascicles are synovial attachments of the posterior horn of the lateral meniscus that extend around the popliteus bursa. The superior fascicle arises from the medial fibers of the popliteus tendon aponeurosis, and the inferior fascicle extends from the meniscus to the tibial margin (Fig. 2). At least one fascicle is visualized in 97% of patients with an intact lateral meniscus, best seen on T2-weighted images [8]. The fascicles control the motion of the lateral meniscus in flexion and extension. Disruption of the fascicles allows increased meniscal movement [6], meniscal subluxation, and even locking of the knee [8]. Along with the popliteus muscle, these structures oppose the forces of the meniscofemoral ligaments [6].

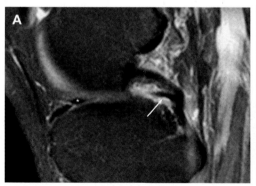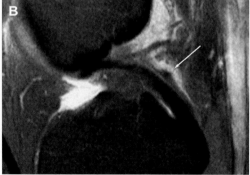

Fig. 1. (*A*) Sagittal gradient echo image of the ligament of Humphrey located anterior to the PCL (*arrow*). Also noted is the anterior or transverse intermeniscal ligament (*asterisk*). (*B*) Sagittal fast spin-echo (FSE) fat-saturated proton density–weighted image of the ligament of Wrisberg, located posterior to the PCL (*arrow*).

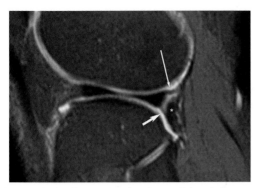

Fig. 2. Sagittal proton density–weighted fat-saturated image of the superior (*thin arrow*) and inferior (*thick arrow*) popliteomeniscal fascicles attaching to the posterior horn of the lateral meniscus, with the popliteus tendon (*asterisk*) in between.

Meniscal variants

Many meniscal variants have been reported. Some of the variants described more commonly include the discoid meniscus, meniscal ossicles, and the meniscal flounce.

The discoid lateral meniscus has a reported incidence of 0.4% to 16.6% and is more common in the Japanese and Korean populations (Fig. 3) [9]. Joint line tenderness is noted in 73%, "snapping" in 49%, and locking of the knee in 21% of patients [10]. The three types of discoid lateral meniscus are complete, incomplete, and the Wrisberg variant. Some investigators include a ring-shaped meniscus as a fourth type [11]. The complete and incomplete types have a firm, normal posterior tibial attachment and are stable [6]. Symptomatic patients who have these types of discoid menisci usually are treated with a partial meniscectomy [12,13]. In contrast, the Wrisberg variant has no posterior coronary or capsular attachments [1,13] and increased T2 signal is present between the meniscus

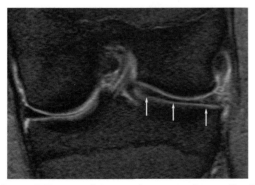

Fig. 3. GRE coronal image demonstrating a discoid lateral meniscus (*arrows*).

and the capsule, simulating a peripheral tear or a fascicular injury [13]. The Wrisberg variant has the most notable symptoms [6], with a "snapping" sensation occurring when the posterior horn moves across the femoral condyle during flexion and extension [13]. Historically, treatment of the Wrisberg variant has been total meniscectomy; however, more recently, some investigators have suggested partial meniscectomy with repair [12,13]. A discoid medial meniscus is much less common, with the incidence reported to be 0.12% to 0.6% [3,14,15].

On MR, the diagnosis of a discoid meniscus is suggested by identifying either meniscal tissue on three continuous sagittal 5-mm-thick slices, or a meniscal body on coronal images greater than 15 mm wide or extending into the intercondylar notch [13,14]. The discoid meniscus has an increased incidence of tears and degeneration, likely caused by its abnormal shape, resulting in increased stress on the meniscus [15–17]. Intrasubstance "grade 2" signal, or abnormal signal not extending to an articular surface, is noted in 24% of discoid menisci and is more common in complete discoid menisci [17]. Typically, this abnormal signal is not considered clinically significant however, in the population with discoid menisci, some investigators report that this intrasubstance signal may be significant clinically [16,17].

Meniscal ossicles are reported in 0.15% of patients and are thought to be either developmental or posttraumatic. These small, ossific foci are found typically in the posterior horn of the medial meniscus and are associated with meniscal tears. They can be asymptomatic, or associated with pain and a sensation of locking, clinically simulating a torn meniscus with a flap component. The ossicle follows the signal of bone marrow on MR [18].

Meniscal flounce is a wavy appearance along the free edge of the meniscus. Previously, meniscal flounce was thought to be identified only at arthroscopy, in the presence of joint fluid with the knee flexed, the tibia rotated externally, and a valgus force applied, exposing the posterior-medial compartment of the knee, or in the setting of an ACL or medial collateral ligament (MCL) tear [19,20]. However, a flounce can be seen without a ligament injury [20]. Recently, the meniscal flounce has been identified with MR imaging when the knee is in 10 degrees of flexion. The flounce completely resolves when the knee is extended maximally, and resolves nearly 50% of the time when the knee is flexed maximally [21]. The flounce can appear truncated on coronal images and can simulate a tear or degeneration. The incidence at MR is reported to be from 0.2% to 6%. A flounce-like appearance can be seen with meniscal tears (Fig. 4) [19,20].

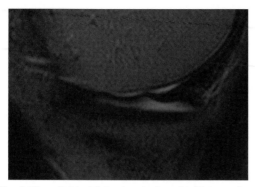

Fig. 4. T2-weighted fat-saturated sagittal image demonstrating a flouncelike appearance to the posterior horn and body of the medial meniscus, in the setting of a meniscal tear.

Meniscal extrusion

Meniscal extrusion is measured from the outer meniscal edge to the proximal tibial margin. Extrusion of the medial meniscus more than 3 mm is considered abnormal (Fig. 5). This degree of extrusion can be seen in patients who have advanced meniscal degeneration, and various types of meniscal tears [22]. Although extrusion of the anterior horn or body of the lateral meniscus sometimes is considered a normal variant [23], others consider extrusion of the lateral meniscus more than 1 mm to be abnormal [24]. Damage to the meniscus and meniscal extrusion can be associated with cartilage abnormalities and likely predisposes to the development of osteoarthritis [22,25].

Tears: etiology

The cause of meniscal tears can be divided into two categories: increased force on a normal meniscus,

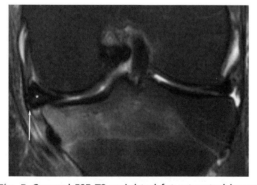

Fig. 5. Coronal FSE T2-weighted fat-saturated image demonstrating medial extrusion (*arrow*) of the body of the medial meniscus (*asterisk*) because of a posterior medial meniscal root tear. Bone contusion is also seen in the medial tibial plateau, with cartilage loss in the medial femoral condyle.

usually resulting in longitudinal or radial tears, and normal forces on a degenerative meniscus, usually producing horizontal tears in the posterior half of the meniscus [26]. Tears are more common in the medial meniscus [1,6], possibly because the medial meniscus is less mobile, and it bears more force during weight-bearing than the lateral meniscus [22,27], with 56% of tears involving the posterior horn of the medial meniscus [28]. Tears isolated to the anterior two thirds of the meniscus are uncommon, representing only 2% of medial and 16% of lateral meniscal tears [29]. Lateral meniscal tears are more common in younger patients (under 30 years old), who have a higher incidence of tears related to sporting events than do older patients. It is likely that this is related to the higher incidence of concomitant ACL tears in this population [30]. The prevalence of meniscal tears increases with age [1], with degenerative tears also more common in older patients [30].

Tears: diagnosis

The diagnosis of a meniscal tear requires high spatial resolution and an optimized signal-to-noise ratio [31], achieved with the use of a dedicated extremity coil, a slice thickness of 3 to 4 mm, a field of view of 16 cm or less, and a matrix size of at least 256 × 192 (frequency and phase). Many MR sequences have been used to evaluate for meniscal tears, and although they vary in other parameters, they all share a short echo time (TE) [32]. The advantages of a short TE include a reduction in scan time, decreased susceptibility and fewer flow artifacts, an ability to acquire more scan slices per sequence, and an improved signal-to-noise ratio.

The most commonly used sequences include spin-echo or fast spin-echo (FSE) proton density with or without fat saturation, T1, and gradient echo (GRE) [32]. Each sequence has investigators who support its use; however, a pooled summary of published articles between 1991 and 2000 reports a sensitivity and specificity with MR imaging of 93% and 88% for medial, and 79% and 95% for lateral meniscal tears [33]. The differences in sensitivity and specificity could be related to the sequences used, observer variation, or sample size [34]. The sensitivity for detecting meniscal tears usually is higher in the medial meniscus, regardless of the technique used [35].

The radiology literature illustrates controversy about the relative accuracies of spin-echo proton density and FSE proton density sequences for detecting meniscal tears [31,36,37]. Conventional proton density spin-echo imaging has a sensitivity and specificity for diagnosing meniscal tears of 88% to 90% and 87% to 90%, respectively

[31,38,39]. The sensitivity and specificity of FSE proton density sequences for diagnosing meniscal tears is 82% to 96% and 84% to 94%, respectively; however, not all of these studies used an echo train length (ETL) less than or equal to five [31,35,40,41]. The overall lower sensitivities reported for the FSE technique are thought to be because of the inherent blurring artifact seen with this technique, which is worsened by a longer ETL and most pronounced with shorter TE sequences [31]. However, the blurring can be reduced by using high-speed gradients and decreasing the ETL and interecho spacing [37]. The addition of fat saturation to FSE and conventional proton density imaging is becoming more common [32,35]. Blackmon and colleagues [42] recently reported a sensitivity of 93% and a specificity of 97% for diagnosing meniscal tears using a fat-saturated conventional spin-echo proton density–weighted sequence, which was 13% more sensitive than a fat-saturated FSE proton density–weighted sequence. Three-dimensional GRE imaging has a sensitivity and specificity for detecting meniscal tears of 87% to 100% and 78% to 94%, respectively [39,43,44], with the best results obtained using an average slice thickness of 3 mm on sagittal and coronal sequences [43]. The limitations of this sequence include a higher signal in normal menisci, compared with spin-echo sequences, and more widespread signal increase in degenerated menisci [39]. This increased meniscal signal can make it difficult to determine if the abnormal signal actually extends to the articular surface, resulting in decreased specificity [44]. The sensitivity and specificity of spin-echo T-1 weighted sequences in detecting meniscal tears is between 77% and 80% and 72% and 98%, respectively [44,45]. Therefore, a sequence with a short TE and an optimized signal-to-noise ratio should be used to evaluate for meniscal pathology, with most using a proton density–weighted sequence.

The normal meniscus has low signal on all MR imaging sequences. On sagittal MR images, the anterior and posterior horns of the lateral meniscus are nearly equal in size, whereas the posterior horn of the medial meniscus is larger than the anterior horn (Fig. 6). The diagnostic criteria for a meniscal tear in a knee without prior meniscal surgery is either an area of abnormal signal within the meniscus on at least one image that extends to the meniscal articular surface, or abnormal morphology of the meniscus [29]. If the abnormal signal extends to the articular surface on two or more images, the sensitivity for a meniscal tear increases from 56% to 94% medially and from 30% to 90% laterally [29]. The sagittal plane is used most commonly to evaluate meniscal pathology; however, studies have reported that the coronal imaging plane improves the detection and characterization of radial, bucket-handle, horizontal, and displaced tears of the meniscal body [46,47], and that the axial plane assists in diagnosing radial, vertical, complex, displaced, and lateral meniscal tears [48,49].

An accurate description of a meniscal tear has become increasingly important, with the emphasis on meniscal preservation and repair [3,28,50,51], because of the known, long-term complications of complete meniscectomy, which include degenerative changes in 21% of cases, patient dissatisfaction in 36% to 40% of cases, marked disability in 30% of cases, and chronic pain in 55% of men and 90% of women [52]. The description should include whether the tear is in the posterior horn, body, or anterior horn, and whether the tear is in the peripheral third of the meniscus (roughly corresponding to the vascularized red zone), the inner two thirds of the meniscus, or both. It should also be stated if the tear is complete, extending from one articular surface to another, or incomplete. The tear should be described as horizontal, vertical (longitudinal, radial, or parrot-beak), or complex.

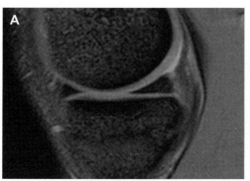 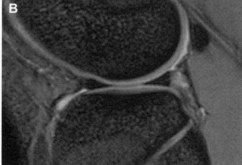

Fig. 6. (*A*) Sagittal GRE image of a normal medial meniscus. (*B*) Sagittal GRE image of a normal lateral meniscus.

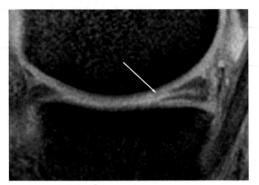

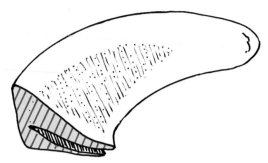

Fig. 8. Horizontal tear.

Fig. 7. Sagittal GRE image demonstrating a horizontal tear (*arrow*) of the posterior horn of the medial meniscus.

The length of the tear is also important because it may determine if the tear is repairable [28]. At arthroscopy, tears can be classified as stable or unstable, with unstable lesions being displaceable into the joint with probing, and more often resected or repaired [53].

Classification of tears

Horizontal tears

Horizontal or cleavage tears are parallel to the tibial plateau and divide the meniscus into upper and lower segments (**Figs. 7 and 8**) [28].

Vertical tears

A vertical longitudinal tear occurs between the circumferential collagen fibers, parallel to the long axis of the meniscus, perpendicular to the tibial plateau, with the tear equidistant from the peripheral edge of the meniscus (**Figs. 9 and 10**) [28].

A vertical radial tear occurs on a plane perpendicular to the long axis of the meniscus and perpendicular to the tibial plateau [28,54,55]. These tears traverse the circumferential collagen fibers, resulting in either two separate pieces of meniscus, or a single portion of meniscus attached to the tibia in only one location [54,55]. The incidence of radial tears is approximately 14% to 15%, with 79% in the posterior horns [3,32,54]. These tears disrupt the ability to distribute the hoop stresses associated with weight-bearing, and usually are not repairable [3]. Partial thickness radial tears can be debrided, but the meniscus is unlikely to regain full function and likely will displace peripherally and allow contact between articular cartilage surfaces, resulting in accelerated degenerative changes [3,32,54,55]. As a result, even small radial tears can have a significant detrimental effect on the function of the meniscus, and can cause pain [3,56]. The prospective detection of radial tears is reported to be as low as 37%; however, using four signs (ghost, cleft, truncated triangle, and marching cleft), the sensitivity for the detection of radial tears is reported to be 89% [3]. A radial tear can have a ghost appearance if there is either an absent section of meniscus or an area of high signal in the shape of the meniscus on a single image that is parallel to the tear. A marching cleft presents most commonly with a radial tear at the junction of the

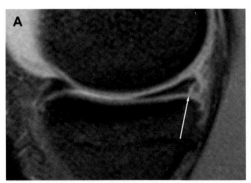

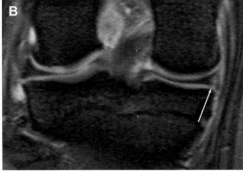

Fig. 9. (*A*) Sagittal GRE image demonstrating a peripheral vertical longitudinal tear (*arrow*) of the posterior horn of the medial meniscus. (*B*) Coronal GRE image demonstrating a peripheral vertical longitudinal tear (*arrow*) of the body of the medial meniscus.

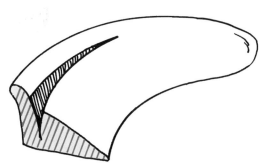

Fig. 10. Vertical longitudinal tear.

posterior horn and body that appears to "move" across the meniscus on successive images. The truncated triangle sign is noted when there is an abrupt truncation of the inner point of the normal meniscus. The cleft sign occurs when there is abnormal signal present in the meniscus perpendicular to the imaging plane (**Figs. 11 and 12**) [3].

Vertical parrot-beak tears are radial at the inner meniscal edge and longitudinal more peripherally within the meniscus [28,55]. These tears are difficult to detect with MR imaging, with reported sensitivities ranging from 0% to 60% (**Fig. 13**) [28].

Complex tears

Complex tears either have two or more tear configurations or are not categorized easily into a certain type of tear [28].

Bucket-handle tears

A bucket-handle tear results when the inner meniscal segment of a longitudinal or oblique tear "flips," most commonly into the intercondylar notch. This often involves the entire meniscus but can involve only the posterior horn and body or a single horn of the meniscus [57]. It is the most common type of displaced "flap" tear, occurring in approximately 10% to 26% of patients [58–60], and is more common medially [47,59–61]. The inner flipped portion of the meniscus can remain intact or it can be disrupted.

The overall sensitivity of MR imaging for bucket-handle fragments is 64% to 94% [47,60–64], with higher sensitivities reported if the tear involves the entire meniscus [47,62]. The MR diagnosis of a bucket-handle tear uses many signs [62,64–66]. The double PCL sign consists of meniscal material in the notch, inferior and parallel to the PCL in the same sagittal plane [57]. It has a sensitivity of 27% to 44% and a specificity of 98% to 100% in detecting bucket-handle tears, and it is noted only in medial bucket-handle tears unless there is an associated ACL tear (**Fig. 14**) [47,60–64]. The fragment in notch sign occurs when a fragment of meniscus is in the notch but not in the same sagittal plane as the PCL (**Fig. 15**). It is seen more often in lateral bucket-handle tears [57], and it has a sensitivity of 60% to 98% and specificity of 73% to 82% for detecting bucket-handle tears [41,47,60,61,63]. The absent bow tie sign is diagnosed when the meniscus body is not identified on at least two adjacent sagittal 4 to 5 mm-thick images. It has a sensitivity of 58% to 98% and a specificity of 62% to 100% for detecting bucket-handle tears [41,59–61,63,64]. False positives with this sign can occur in children or small adults, in degenerative menisci, in radial tears, and with postsurgical changes [32,61]. False negatives can occur in bucket-handle tears of discoid menisci [61]. A truncated meniscus on coronal images is reported in up to 65% of bucket-handle tears [61,64]. The disproportional posterior horn

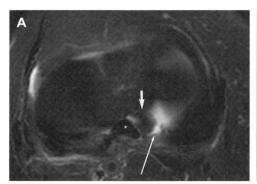

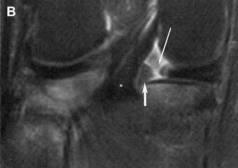

Fig. 11. (A) FSE T2-weighted fat-saturated axial image demonstrating a radial tear (*thin arrow*) of the posterior horn of the medial meniscus near the posterior meniscal root attachment (*thick arrow*). Note the proximity of the PCL (*asterisk*) to the posterior root attachment of the posterior horn of the medial meniscus. (B) FSE T2-weighted fat-saturated coronal image demonstrating a radial tear (*thin arrow*) in the posterior horn of the medial meniscus with the cleft sign. The posterior medial meniscal root is intact (*thick arrow*). Note the proximity of the PCL (*asterisk*) to the posterior root attachment of the posterior horn of the medial meniscus.

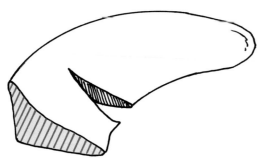

Fig. 12. Vertical radial tear.

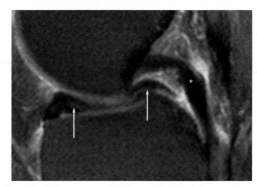

Fig. 14. FSE proton density–weighted fat-saturated sagittal sequence demonstrating a bucket-handle tear of the medial meniscus. The double PCL sign is present, with the flipped fragment of the medial meniscal body (*arrows*) located anterior to the PCL (*asterisk*) within the intercondylar notch.

sign is present when there is a larger posterior horn on sagittal images closer to the root attachment than peripherally, presumably because of a centrally displaced fragment of the more peripheral posterior horn. This sign has a sensitivity of approximately 28% for bucket-handle tears [60,63]. A quadruple cruciate sign can be observed if there are medial and lateral bucket-handle meniscal tears, with both fragments displaced into the notch (Fig. 16) [67].

The flipped meniscus sign, which occurs when the fragment is flipped anteriorly adjacent to the ipsilateral anterior horn [57], is noted in 44% to 61% of medial and 29% to 39% of lateral bucket-handle tears [61,62]. The anterior horn should not measure greater than 6 mm in height; if it does, this should be considered. The double anterior horn sign is the same as the flipped meniscus sign; however, two separate "anterior horns" are identified (Fig. 17). Usually, the flipped meniscus and double anterior horn signs are associated with intercondylar meniscal displacement [57].

Flap tear with displacement

A flap tear or a displaced flap tear is a term that is used often to describe a short-segment, horizontal meniscal tear with fragments either displaced into the notch or into the superior or inferior gutters

(Fig. 18) [41,57]. These tears are unstable [41] and are important to recognize and describe, especially if the flap of meniscal tissue extends into the inferior gutter because this is a difficult area for the surgeon to visualize (Fig. 19) [58]. The failure to identify and treat recess fragments is a known cause of poor outcome after meniscal resection [41]. This tear can be suspected when the normal rectangular meniscus is not identified on the most peripheral sagittal image, and meniscal tissue is noted inferior to the body segment [58]. The coronal images are the most useful in confirming the inferiorly displaced meniscal tissue.

Free fragments

Free fragment displacement is rare, occurring in 0.2% of symptomatic meniscal lesions [57].

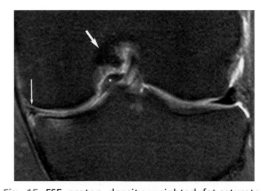

Fig. 15. FSE proton density–weighted fat-saturated coronal sequence demonstrating a bucket-handle tear of the medial meniscus, with a portion of the body of the medial meniscus located in the intercondylar notch (*asterisk*) beneath the PCL (*thick arrow*) and adjacent to the ACL. Note the remainder of the body of the medial meniscus is truncated (*thin arrow*).

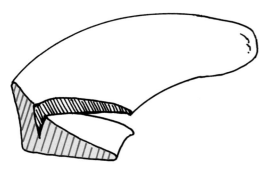

Fig. 13. Vertical parrot-beak tear.

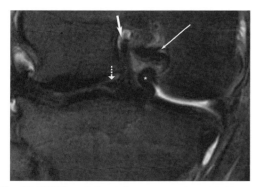

Fig. 16. FSE T2-weighted fat-saturated coronal image demonstrating bucket-handle tears of both menisci, with fragments from both meniscal bodies flipped into the intercondylar notch. The fragment of the medial meniscus (*asterisk*) is inferior to the PCL (*thin arrow*) and the fragment of the body of the lateral meniscus (*dotted arrow*) is adjacent to the ACL (*thick arrow*), producing the "quadruple cruciate sign."

Root tears

A root tear occurs at the tibial attachment or "root" of the meniscus, and it has been described only posteriorly (**Fig. 20**) [24]. Actually, this type of tear was described by Tuckman and colleagues [55] but was called a full thickness radial tear at, or adjacent to, the tibial attachments. Studies have described an association between extrusion of the medial meniscus, medial compartment arthritis, and posterior-medial meniscal root tears [24,55].

A root tear is reportedly a difficult tear to diagnose because meniscal tissue is noted only on one side of the tear. The diagnosis is easier to make medially because of the close anatomic relationship between the posterior horn of the meniscus and the tibial attachment of the PCL. Normally, on 3-mm sagittal images, the meniscus should be seen on

the image medial to the PCL attachment; otherwise, a root tear is suspected and the coronal images can confirm [55]. Meniscal extrusion is more pronounced and nearly four times as common with medial, as opposed to lateral, meniscal root tears [24]. Lateral meniscal root tears are diagnosed when the posterior horn of the lateral meniscus does not cover the most medial aspect of the posterior lateral tibial plateau on at least one coronal image [55]. In the setting of an ACL tear, the lateral meniscal root is torn more than three times as often as the medial root, with lateral meniscal extrusion greater than 1 mm present in 23% of patients who have lateral root tears and in 2% of those who have intact lateral meniscal roots. All patients who had meniscal extrusion but intact roots had another type of meniscal tear, with 60% having radial or complex tears. Extrusion was noted nearly four times as often in lateral meniscal root tears if the meniscofemoral ligaments were absent [24].

Meniscal tears in the setting of anterior cruciate ligament tears

In the setting of an acute ACL injury, the lateral meniscus is torn twice as often as the medial meniscus, with approximately one half representing peripheral longitudinal tears most commonly located in the posterior horn of the lateral meniscus [68,69]. Displaced meniscal tears are also more common in this setting [38]. The sensitivity for diagnosing meniscal tears is decreased in these patients primarily because of failure to detect lateral meniscal tears (**Fig. 21**) [68,69].

In ACL-deficient knees, the increased shear forces on the less mobile posterior horn of the medial meniscus may account for the increased rate of medial meniscal tears [1,70], which possibly is related to

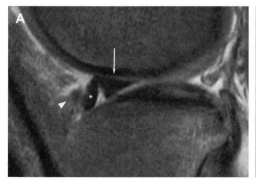

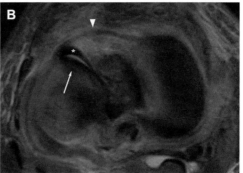

Fig. 17. (*A*) Sagittal FSE proton density–weighted fat-saturated image demonstrating a tear of the lateral meniscus, with the fragment of the body (*long arrow*) flipped adjacent to the anterior horn (*asterisk*). Note the anterior transverse intermeniscal ligament (*arrowhead*). (*B*) Axial FSE proton density–weighted fat-saturated image demonstrating flipped fragment of lateral meniscus body (*long arrow*) adjacent to the anterior horn of the lateral meniscus (*asterisk*). Note bowing of the anterior transverse intermeniscal ligament (*arrowhead*).

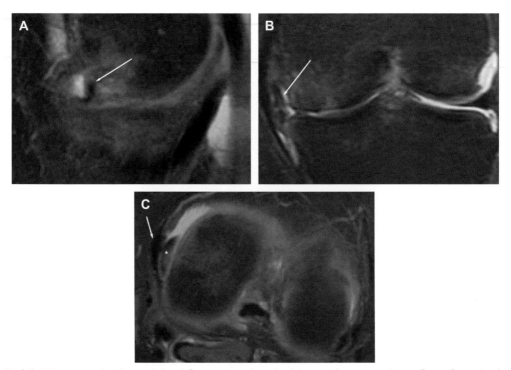

Fig. 18. (A) FSE proton density–weighted fat-saturated sagittal image demonstrating a flap of meniscal tissue (*arrow*) extending from the anterior horn body junction of the medial meniscus into the superior recess medially. (B) Coronal short tau inversion recovery (STIR) image demonstrating the flap of meniscal tissue (*arrow*) extending into the superior aspect of the medial recess. Medial compartment chondromalacia is also noted. (C) FSE proton density–weighted fat-saturated axial image demonstrating a flap of meniscal tissue (*asterisk*) deep to the MCL (*arrow*) and superficial to the medial femoral condyle in the superior aspect of the medial recess.

the increased posterior translation of the femur in relation to the tibia with flexion in ACL-deficient knees [70]. These tears are often less amenable to repair; therefore, early ACL repair in certain populations (athletes and manual laborers) should be considered [1].

Meniscal pitfalls

Seventy percent of false-positive MR imaging findings occur in the posterior horns of the menisci, which are the most difficult areas to evaluate at arthroscopy [29,52,71,72]. The standard arthroscopic technique for evaluating the posterior horn of the medial meniscus is to probe the tibial surface while compressing the femoral surface [52]. Because evaluation of the meniscal gutters is also difficult, the accuracy of arthroscopy for diagnosing meniscal tears is 69% to 98%, depending on the arthroscopist and the location and type of tear [71]. Therefore, some of the cases considered false positives on MR imaging might, in fact, represent false negatives on arthroscopy.

False positives can also occur with healed meniscal tears or postoperative menisci, in which

abnormal signal extending to the surface remains on standard MR imaging sequences [29,52]. False positives because of magic angle phenomenon on sequences with a TE less than 37 can also occur in the posterior horn of the lateral meniscus because of the central upsloping of the meniscus [73]. Truncation artifact can also be a cause of false positives;

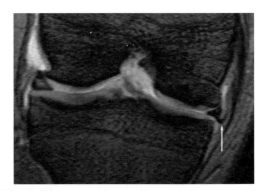

Fig. 19. GRE coronal image demonstrating truncation of the body of the medial meniscus (truncated triangle sign), with the flap of meniscal tissue flipped under the meniscus into the inferior recess medially (*arrow*).

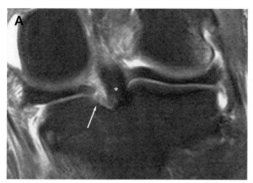
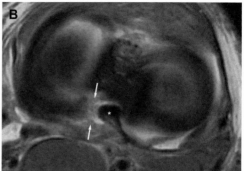

Fig. 20. (A) FSE proton density–weighted fat-saturated coronal image demonstrating a tear of the posterior medial meniscal root (*arrow*). Note the tibial attachment of the PCL (*asterisk*). (B) Axial FSE proton density–weighted fat-saturated image demonstrating a tear of the posterior medial meniscal root (*arrows*). Note the proximity to normal tibial attachment of PCL (*asterisk*).

however, the use of a matrix of at least 192 × 256 minimizes this artifact such that it is seen rarely today [74]. Radially orientated collagen "tie" fibers, which have linear intermediate signal within the meniscus, and myxoid degeneration can also simulate tears [4]. Abnormal signal having a speckled or spotty appearance on T1 and proton density images can occur in the anterior horn of the lateral meniscus near the central attachment on the most central sagittal images [32], thought to be caused by high signal striations from the ACL fibers [75]. Sometimes, the transverse intermeniscal ligament can simulate a tear in the anterior horns of either menisci (Fig. 22) [5,76]. The lateral inferior genicular artery can simulate a tear of the lateral meniscus, and the normal concavity of the peripheral aspect of the meniscus can mimic a horizontal tear on peripheral sagittal images caused by a volume-averaging artifact [76]. The meniscal attachments of the meniscofemoral ligaments can simulate a tear in the posterior horn of the lateral meniscus [77]. The popliteus tendon adjacent to the posterior horn of the lateral meniscus can also be a source of error because of fluid tracking along the intra-articular portion of the tendon [8,76]. The medial and lateral oblique meniscomeniscal ligaments and [78] the anterior meniscofemoral ligament of the medial meniscus [79] can also simulate tears. However, following these structures on multiple images, evaluating the meniscus in different imaging planes, and having a thorough understanding of the anatomy often can prevent these errors.

Meniscal contusion can demonstrate abnormal amorphous or globular meniscal signal that contacts an articular surface but is less discrete and less well defined than the signal associated with a tear and intrasubstance degeneration, respectively. All patients have adjacent bone contusions and most have ACL tears. The abnormal signal can resolve over time [80].

The diagnostic accuracy of MR imaging for meniscal tears decreases in patients who have chondrocalcinosis because the calcium deposits may demonstrate high signal on T1-weighted, intermediate-weighted, and short tau inversion recovery (STIR) sequences [81]. Reviewing radiographs can alert the radiologist to the chondrocalcinosis. In addition, most meniscal tears are more linear than the signal abnormalities seen with chondrocalcinosis; however, there is overlap [32].

Common false negatives at MR imaging include small meniscal tears and abnormalities involving the meniscal free edge [52].

Meniscocapsular separation

Meniscocapsular separation occurs when the meniscus detaches from the capsular attachments [82], which is more common medially and usually is associated with other injuries [83]. The medial capsuloligamentous structures can be thought of

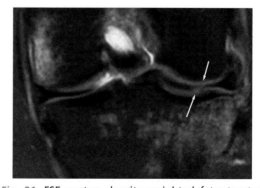

Fig. 21. FSE proton density–weighted fat-saturated coronal image demonstrating a subtle area of abnormal signal, representing a meniscal tear, extending to the articular surfaces (*arrows*) of the posterior horn of the lateral meniscus in a patient who had an ACL tear. The meniscal tear was not diagnosed prospectively.

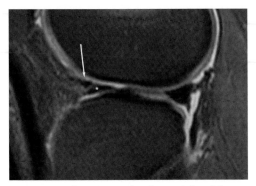

Fig. 22. Spin-echo proton density–weighted fat-saturated sagittal image demonstrating the anterior (transverse) intermeniscal ligament (*arrow*) simulating a tear of the anterior horn of the lateral meniscus (*asterisk*). A similar finding was present at the junction with the anterior horn of the medial meniscus.

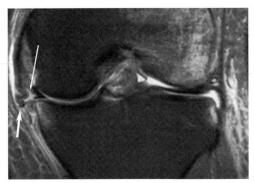

Fig. 23. FSE proton density–weighted fat-saturated coronal image demonstrating fluid signal and widening (*thin arrow*) between the medial edge of the body of the medial meniscus and the MCL, consistent with meniscocapsular separation. Note the complete disruption of the tibial attachment of the MCL (*thick arrow*).

as three layers, from superficial to deep: layer 1: crural fascia; layer 2: superficial portion of the MCL; and layer 3: capsule and deep portion of the MCL [84]. The medial meniscus is attached to the femur by way of the meniscofemoral ligament, and to the tibia by way of the coronary (meniscotibial) ligament, which are extensions of the deep fibers of the MCL [84].

Meniscocapsular separation is evaluated best on coronal and sagittal T1- or proton density–weighted sequences for anatomy, and fat-saturated T2-weighted or STIR sequences for pathology [84]. Signs that have been described in meniscocapsular separation include displacement of the meniscus relative to the tibial margin, extension of the tear into the superior or inferior corner of the peripheral meniscus, and an irregular outer margin of the meniscus body on coronal images. Additional signs include increased distance between the meniscus and the MCL, or fluid between the meniscus and the MCL [83,84]. A study by Rubin and colleagues [82] reported a positive predictive value of only 9% for the MR diagnosis of medial meniscocapsular separation using these signs; however, the positive predictive value improved to 17% if the surgery was performed within 2 weeks of the MR imaging, likely because these injuries occur in an area with an extensive blood supply and many heal conservatively [82–84]. Overall, the presence of perimeniscal fluid and an irregular meniscal outline are the best predictors of meniscocapsular separation (Fig. 23) [84].

Findings associated with meniscal tears

The use of indirect signs to increase the accuracy for the detection of lateral meniscal tears has been

reported [85]. A torn or absent superior popliteomeniscal fascicle was noted in 31% of patients with, and 4% without, lateral meniscal tears [86]. Presumptive subarticular stress reactions of the knee are characterized by an edema-like pattern in the subarticular marrow, which encompasses a focal, linear, or curvilinear low-signal area. Of these patients, 76% have a meniscal tear in the same compartment, with 53% being either radial or root tears. These lesions occur in a much older population and likely are caused by radial or root tears that predispose the knee to increased stress which, in an older population, results in insufficiency-type lesions [87]. The lesions have a similar appearance to spontaneous osteonecrosis of the knee, which is a reported complication of radial tears, especially in older patients with large body habitus [55], and in patients who have had a prior medial meniscectomy or degenerative medial meniscal tears [88,89].

Subchondral bone contusions involving the posterior margin of the medial tibial plateau in patients who have ACL tears are associated with posterior horn medial meniscal tears in 64% of patients and meniscocapsular separation/injury in 56% of patients, with either one of the two injuries noted in 96% of the patients. The mechanism is thought to be a contrecoup impaction injury, with 62% of the medial meniscal tears in the far peripheral 20% of the meniscus. Lateral meniscal tears were also noted in 36% of these patients [90].

Meniscal cysts

Meniscal cysts are identified on 4% to 6% of knee MR examinations, are located twice as often medially, and may be lobulated or septated in appearance [32,91,92]. The cysts can be confined within the meniscus (intermeniscal) or can extend into the adjacent soft tissue (perimeniscal), with the latter more common [93]. The most widely accepted cause of a meniscal cyst is extension of fluid through a meniscal tear [91], with 57% noted in horizontal cleavage and 33% in complex tears with a horizontal component [91,93]. Medially, the cysts are adjacent to the posterior horn, with anterior extension adjacent to the body in 74% of cases (Fig. 24) [91,92]. Laterally, the cysts are adjacent to the anterior horn, with posterior extension adjacent to the body in 54% of cases. Direct communication between the meniscal cyst and the meniscal tear is noted in 98% of cases. Lateral meniscal cysts more often present as palpable masses, likely because of the thinner, overlying, lateral soft tissues [91]. Occasionally, a posterior horn medial meniscal tear can produce a cyst that extends centrally within the joint adjacent to the posterior central aspect of the PCL or surrounding the PCL, simulating a ganglion [93]. Treatment of meniscal cysts involves decompression of the cyst and repair or resection of the tear, usually from an exclusively intra-articular approach [91]. Therefore, detection of an associated tear is important; it may alter therapy because perimeniscal cysts without an underlying tear often are treated percutaneously. The cysts can be symptomatic with or without a tear [32].

MR imaging field strength

Several studies suggest similar accuracy for diagnosing meniscal tears with 0.2 T and 1.5 T MR imaging, although some controversy remains [94,95]. Undoubtedly, scanning time is longer at lower field strengths, 15 minutes longer at 0.2 T than at 1.5 T in one article [95]. A higher confidence for diagnosing meniscal tears at 1.5 T, compared with 0.2 T, has

been reported, with the exception of the posterior horn of the lateral meniscus, likely because of the inherent increased signal-to-noise ratio at 1.5 T [96].

Treatment

The four main options for treating meniscal tears are complete meniscectomy, partial meniscectomy, meniscal repair, and conservative treatment without meniscal surgery [28]. The treatment of meniscal lesions depends on many factors, including the type, location, and size of the tear. Initially, meniscal lesions were treated with complete meniscectomy because the importance of the meniscus and its function were not understood well [97,98]. Unfortunately, complete meniscectomy has been shown to result in accelerated cartilage loss and the development of osteoarthritis [1,4,51,97–100]. Partial meniscectomy is less damaging to the joint and is preferred to a complete meniscectomy in patients who have unstable tears [1], when a primary meniscal repair is not possible [28]. Preservation of as much of the meniscus as possible, especially the outer third, and removing only unstable tissue, is the desired result; usually, however, some stable tissue is resected to approximate the original meniscal shape, in an attempt to reduce the inevitable increased stress on the remaining meniscal tissue [97]. Many studies have shown progressive, long-term wear on the joint after partial meniscectomy, with a declining number of patients reporting excellent or good results over time [99]. This result is possibly because of the altered biomechanics of the meniscus, with the decreased ability of the meniscus to transmit hoop stresses, thereby resulting in increased stress on the remaining meniscus, additional tears, and accelerated degenerative change [101]. As a result, meniscal repair has

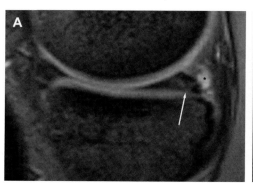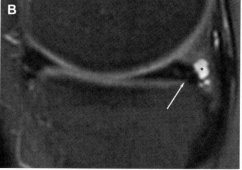

Fig. 24. (*A*) GRE sagittal image demonstrating a perimeniscal cyst (*asterisk*) adjacent to the posterior horn of the medial meniscus, with the tear (*arrow*) extending to the cyst. (*B*) FSE proton density–weighted fat-saturated sagittal image demonstrating a perimeniscal cyst (*asterisk*) adjacent to the posterior horn of the medial meniscus, with the tear (*arrow*) extending to the cyst.

become more common, to maintain as much of the normal biomechanical function of the meniscus as possible [28,50,102]. Repairable meniscal tears usually are unstable, peripheral, longitudinal, or oblique tears. Radial, horizontal, or complex tears usually are not amenable to repair [28,102]. After meniscal repair, patients are kept non- or partially weight bearing for several weeks, in contrast to partial meniscectomy, after which patients can resume full weight bearing much more quickly [28]. Healing usually takes 4 months and once the tear heals, patients are usually asymptomatic. The long-term success of meniscal repairs varies from 67% to 92%, depending on the type and location of the tear [1]. Factors that predispose to a favorable repair outcome include surgery within 8 weeks of injury, patient age under 30 years, tear length less than 2.5 cm, a peripheral tear, a lateral meniscus tear, and concomitant ACL reconstruction [1,28]. Therefore, an accurate description of meniscal tears as repairable and irreparable has significant clinical implications, especially for athletes, because continued stress on a potentially repairable tear might make it irreparable [28].

Tears in the peripheral, vascularized portion of the meniscus can heal from an ingrowth of capillaries and eventually resemble fibrocartilage [26,51,97]. Many of these tears may heal spontaneously and not require arthroscopy [51,52]. Longitudinal tears greater than 7 to 10 mm in length, especially post-traumatic vertical peripheral tears, may heal if they are stable [97]. Some surgeons may not operate on horizontal or oblique partial-thickness tears [103], and if a partial meniscectomy is performed on one of these tears, only the unstable portions may be removed, leaving a horizontal defect extending to the articular surface [97]. In patients who have both lateral meniscal and ACL tears, the tear is typically in the periphery of the posterior horn or at the posterior root, and it is important to report if the tear extends anterior to the popliteus hiatus because tears posterior to the hiatus will not always be repaired.

Autologous meniscal transplantation has become more common, especially in younger patients who have had prior partial meniscectomy or who have irreparable meniscal tears [97]. Other appropriate candidates are those with mild to moderate single-compartment cartilage degeneration, those with progressive loss of meniscal tissue but an appropriate varus/valgus alignment, and those having an ACL repair in which a meniscal transplant might improve stabilization [104,105]. Often, meniscal transplantation is performed concomitantly with other procedures, including cruciate ligament or cartilage repair and high-tibial osteotomies [105]. The procedure involves attaching the allograft to the tibia with bone plugs and then suturing the allograft to the capsule. Some reports indicate that MR imaging may be helpful in determining the appropriate size of the meniscal transplant [106]; however, other studies suggest radiographs are nearly as accurate as MR [107]. MR imaging is helpful preoperatively to evaluate the integrity of the ligaments and cartilage [102].

Postoperative imaging

Postoperative imaging of the meniscus is complicated. The standard criteria for a tear has limited diagnostic usefulness when diagnosing a tear at the site of meniscal repair or partial resection, with sensitivity up to 100% but specificity as low as 23% [50,51,100], because of either intermeniscal granulation tissue, which can have abnormal T1-weighted or proton density signal extending to the meniscal surface in the repaired or healing meniscus, or the possible "conversion" of grade 1 or 2 intrameniscal signal to an apparent tear or grade 3 signal by performing a partial meniscectomy [51,97,108]. This appearance can persist for years after a repair [102]. The specificity for diagnosing a tear in this population can be improved if fluid signal is noted in the meniscus on T2-weighted images or if a displaced meniscal fragment is identified (Fig. 25) [97]. The exception may be in the early postoperative period (<12 weeks) when scar tissue at the repair site may demonstrate increased T2-weighted signal [100]. Therefore, the use of gadolinium with either direct or indirect arthrography to detect residual or recurrent tears has been proposed.

Indirect arthrography involves the acquisition of MR images 10 to 20 minutes after the intravenous injection of gadolinium (usually 0.1 mmol/kg). Synovial excretion of contrast occurs, and a tear can be diagnosed if gadolinium signal is noted in the meniscus. However, the natural appearance of a meniscal repair on indirect MR arthrography is abnormal signal extending to the articular surface, seen in 90% of patients, which is seen in only 25% of patients with conventional MR imaging [109]. Therefore, false positives occur because granulation tissue or scar may enhance [97].

Direct arthrography involves the intra-articular injection of approximately 20 mL of a gadolinium-saline mixture (1:150 solution) into the knee. The patient should then walk on the knee before the MR imaging, to force the contrast into meniscal clefts. The extension of contrast into the meniscus diagnoses a recurrent or residual tear (Fig. 26). A healed or repaired tear has abnormal intermeniscal signal without gadolinium extending into the meniscus (Fig. 27) [97]. Even though the intra-articular injection of gadolinium is considered

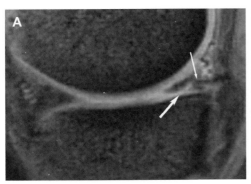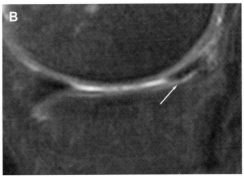

Fig. 25. (A) GRE sagittal image demonstrating abnormal signal extending to the articular surface (*thick arrow*) of the posterior horn of the medial meniscus after meniscal repair. Note focal area of susceptibility artifact from meniscal repair (*thin arrow*). Arthroscopy confirmed a recurrent tear. (B) FSE proton density–weighted fat-saturated sagittal image demonstrating abnormal (fluid) signal extending to the articular surface (*arrow*) of the posterior horn of the medial meniscus after meniscal repair. Arthroscopy confirmed a recurrent tear.

an off-label use by the US Food and Drug Administration, direct arthrography has three advantages over the other methods of evaluating the postoperative meniscus. These advantages include the lower viscosity of gadolinium compared with synovial fluid, making it more likely to extend into a tear; contrast distension of the joint, making fluid more likely to extend into a tear; and the inherent higher signal-to-noise ratio of the T1-weighted sequences used to evaluate the gadolinium contrast [108].

Several investigators report an overall accuracy in detecting recurrent tears of 62% to 77% with conventional MR imaging, 93% with indirect arthrography, and 88% to 92% using direct MR arthrography [108,110,111]. In contrast, White and colleagues reported accuracies of 80%, 81%, and 85% in the diagnosis of recurrent meniscal tears using conventional MR imaging, indirect MR arthrography, and direct MR arthrography, respectively. Although the detection of recurrent tears with direct MR arthrography was minimally higher in White and colleagues [50] study, it did not reach statistical significance. The consensus is that in patients with resection of less than 25% of the meniscus, conventional MR imaging is as accurate as MR arthrography, and that the criteria to diagnose a tear in these patients should be the same as that used for a meniscus without prior surgery [50,110,112]. However, in patients with resection of more than 25% of the meniscus, Applegate and colleagues [110] results demonstrate an accuracy for detecting recurrent tears of only 63% using conventional MR, and an accuracy of 89% using direct MR arthrography. Similar findings led Magee and colleagues [112] to conclude that, in the absence of chondral injuries, avascular necrosis, or severe degenerative changes, patients who have undergone

meniscal repair or those who have had more than 25% of the meniscus resected should have direct MR arthrography performed to detect recurrent tears, because abnormal signal may persist in the meniscus after surgery. In addition, if more than one third of the meniscus is removed, the meniscus can demonstrate surface irregularity on conventional MR images but be found normal at second-look arthroscopy. This surface irregularity can simulate a tear [97] or obscure a recurrent or residual tear [113]. In contrast, menisci with less than one third resection do not demonstrate as much irregularity [113]. Magee and colleagues [101] also reported more than twice the incidence of radial tears in patients who had had prior partial meniscectomies, compared with those without prior surgery, likely because of altered biomechanics.

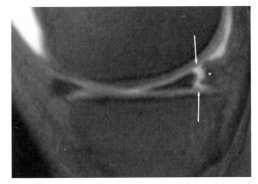

Fig. 26. T1-weighted fat-saturated sagittal MR arthrogram demonstrating a new peripheral vertical longitudinal tear (*arrows*) of the posterior horn of the medial meniscus. Note peripheral aspect of the posterior horn of the medial meniscus (*asterisk*).

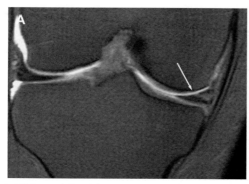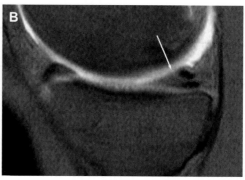

Fig. 27. (A) T1-weighted fat-saturated coronal image from a direct MR arthrogram in a patient following meniscal repair demonstrating abnormal signal extending to the superior surface of the body of the medial meniscus *(arrow)*. No gadolinium extends into this area, confirming a healed meniscal repair. *(B)* T1-weighted fat-saturated sagittal image from a direct MR arthrogram in a patient following meniscal repair demonstrating abnormal signal extending to the superior surface of the body of the medial meniscus *(arrow)*. No gadolinium extends into this area, confirming a healed meniscal repair.

The role of MR imaging in evaluating meniscal allografts is not defined clearly [97]. GRE sequences should be avoided and FSE imaging should be considered instead, because extensive susceptibility artifacts associated with meniscal transplantation and the often associated procedures, including ACL repair or high tibial osteotomy, invariably are present [104]. Reports of MR imaging follow-up are limited, but several suggest that MR findings may not correlate with clinical results; however, these findings were performed on low-intermediate strength magnets and only small numbers of patients were evaluated [114,115]. Other studies, at least one performed on a high-field strength magnet, have suggested that MR can provide information about the position of the meniscus, the meniscal anchors, the meniscocapsular junction, meniscal degeneration, and cartilage defects [104,116]. Most meniscal transplants demonstrate focal degeneration in the posterior horn, associated with moderate to severe cartilage degeneration. As a result, performing pretransplant MR imaging to access for cartilage changes, which might result in a less favorable outcome, should be considered [104]. Increased T2-weighted signal is noted occasionally at the periphery of the transplanted meniscus and is considered normal, likely related to cellular ingrowth or revascularization [116]. Abnormal signal extending to the articular surface of the allograft is noted in 59% of the transplants after 10 or more years; however, the signal is stable in 82% of the allografts and was noted initially on the 1-year posttransplant follow-up MR imaging [114]. Partial extrusion of the allograft is noted in 70% of cases, with progressive extrusion noted in 59% [114,117]. Lack of progressive cartilage loss is reported in just under one half of the viable meniscal transplanted knees [114]. Findings suggestive of meniscal transplant failure include meniscal-fragmentation, progressive articular cartilage loss, and peripheral meniscal extrusion (Fig. 28) [102].

Future imaging: ultrashort echo time imaging, parallel imaging, and 3 Tesla

Ultrashort TE imaging (TEs of 0.08–0.2 ms) is a technique in which the normal meniscus demonstrates increased signal and tears have decreased signal, and is performed best without fat suppression [118]. In contrast to fat-suppressed T1 and Fast Low Angle Shot (FLASH) sequences with intravenous gadolinium, which cannot differentiate between the vascular and avascular zones of the meniscus [4], contrast administration on ultrashort TE images can make this differentiation [118,119].

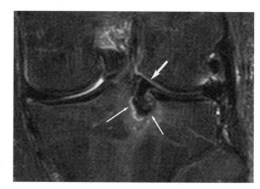

Fig. 28. FSE T2-weighted fat-saturated coronal image of a lateral meniscal transplant. Tunnel *(thin arrows)* for posterior root *(thick arrow)* adjacent to lateral tibial spine.

The full benefit of this sequence has not been described yet.

Parallel imaging reportedly provides a comparable performance to FSE proton density imaging using an ETL of five for meniscal lesions, with nearly a 50% reduction in scan time [120]. No appreciable difference in the sensitivity, specificity, and accuracy for detecting meniscal tears using FSE techniques with and without parallel imaging has been reported [121].

Higher diagnostic confidence is reported with 1.5 T imaging, as opposed to 0.2 T imaging, for the diagnosis of meniscal tears, probably because of the inherent increased signal-to-noise ratio at 1.5 T [33,96]. One could suppose that with 3 T imaging, the confidence and accuracy of detecting meniscal lesions will continue to increase. Three tesla imaging, using FSE proton density–weighted sequences with an ETL of six in the sagittal plane, 2- to 3-mm slice thickness, and a total acquisition time of approximately 20 minutes, has an overall sensitivity and specificity for meniscal tears of 95% to 96% and 92% to 97%, respectively according to McGee and colleagues and Ramnath and colleagues [122,123]. However, Craig, and colleagues [124] reported a sensitivity and specificity of 100% and 83% for medial, and 67% and 97% for lateral meniscus tears with an overall sensitivity and specificity for meniscal tears of 90% and 92% respectively. Further studies are required to determine the true impact of 3 T in evaluating the meniscus, but these results compare favorably to results at 1.5 T using conventional spin-echo sequences.

Summary

MR imaging is the preferred imaging modality for evaluating meniscal pathology, with high accuracy reported in most studies. Achieving this high accuracy requires a thorough knowledge of the anatomy of the meniscus and perimeniscal structures, an understanding of normal variants and interpretive pitfalls, an awareness of the common findings associated with meniscal tears, and an understanding of the diagnostic criteria for a meniscal tear. In patients who have partial meniscal resection or meniscal repair, diagnosing a recurrent tear is more complicated, and the addition of T2 fat-saturated coronal and sagittal sequences to a routine conventional MR protocol is recommended. If there is knowledge of resection of more than 25% of the meniscus or a meniscal repair, most advocate the use of direct MR arthrography. Recent developments in the area of 3 T and faster imaging techniques are not yet evaluated fully, but offer promise for accurate meniscal evaluation with even shorter scan times.

Acknowledgments

I would like to thank D. Laurie Persson and K. Fox for their invaluable assistance in the preparation of the figures and manuscript, respectively.

References

[1] Rath E, Richmond JC. The menisci: basic science and advances in treatment. Br J Sports Med 2000;34(4):252–7.

[2] Fithian DC, Kelly MA, Mow VC. Material properties and structure-function relationships in the menisci. Clin Orthop Relat Res Mar 1990;(252):19–31.

[3] Harper KW, Helms CA, Lambert HS 3rd, et al. Radial meniscal tears: significance, incidence, and MR appearance. AJR Am J Roentgenol 2005;185(6):1429–34.

[4] Hauger O, Frank LR, Boutin RD, et al. Characterization of the "red zone" of knee meniscus: MR imaging and histologic correlation. Radiology 2000;217(1):193–200.

[5] Aydingoz U, Kaya A, Atay OA, et al. MR imaging of the anterior intermeniscal ligament: classification according to insertion sites. Eur Radiol 2002;12(4):824–9.

[6] Gupte CM, Bull AM, Thomas RD, et al. A review of the function and biomechanics of the meniscofemoral ligaments. Arthroscopy 2003;19(2): 161–71.

[7] Lee BY, Jee WH, Kim JM, et al. Incidence and significance of demonstrating the meniscofemoral ligament on MRI. Br J Radiol 2000; 73(867):271–4.

[8] Johnson RL, De Smet AA. MR visualization of the popliteomeniscal fascicles. Skeletal Radiol 1999;28(10):561–6.

[9] Samoto N, Kozuma M, Tokuhisa T, et al. Diagnosis of discoid lateral meniscus of the knee on MR imaging. Magn Reson Imaging 2002; 20(1):59–64.

[10] Rao PS, Rao SK, Paul R. Clinical, radiologic, and arthroscopic assessment of discoid lateral meniscus. Arthroscopy 2001;17(3):275–7.

[11] Arnold MP, Van Kampen A. Symptomatic ring-shaped lateral meniscus. Arthroscopy 2000; 16(8):852–4.

[12] Asik M, Sen C, Taser OF, et al. Discoid lateral meniscus: diagnosis and results of arthroscopic treatment. Knee Surg Sports Traumatol Arthrosc 2003;11(2):99–104.

[13] Singh K, Helms CA, Jacobs MT, et al. MRI appearance of Wrisberg variant of discoid lateral meniscus. AJR Am J Roentgenol 2006; 187(2):384–7.

[14] Tachibana Y, Yamazaki Y, Ninomiya S. Discoid medial meniscus. Arthroscopy 2003;19(7): E12–8.

[15] Rohren EM, Kosarek FJ, Helms CA. Discoid lateral meniscus and the frequency of meniscal tears. Skeletal Radiol 2001;30(6):316–20.

[16] Ryu KN, Kim IS, Kim EJ, et al. MR imaging of tears of discoid lateral menisci. AJR Am J Roentgenol 1998;171(4):963–7.

[17] Araki Y, Ashikaga R, Fujii K, et al. MR imaging of meniscal tears with discoid lateral meniscus. Eur J Radiol 1998;27(2):153–60.

[18] Schnarkowski P, Tirman PF, Fuchigami KD, et al. Meniscal ossicle: radiographic and MR imaging findings. Radiology 1995;196(1):47–50.

[19] Yu JS, Cosgarea AJ, Kaeding CC, et al. Meniscal flounce MR imaging. Radiology 1997;203(2):513–5.

[20] Kim BH, Seol HY, Jung HS, et al. Meniscal flounce on MR: correlation with arthroscopic or surgical findings. Yonsei Med J 2000;41(4):507–11.

[21] Park JS, Ryu KN, Yoon KH. Meniscal flounce on knee MRI: correlation with meniscal locations after positional changes. AJR Am J Roentgenol 2006;187(2):364–70.

[22] Costa CR, Morrison WB, Carrino JA. Medial meniscus extrusion on knee MRI: is extent associated with severity of degeneration or type of tear? AJR Am J Roentgenol 2004;183(1):17–23.

[23] Miller TT, Staron RB, Feldman F, et al. Meniscal position on routine MR imaging of the knee. Skeletal Radiol 1997;26(7):424–7.

[24] Brody JM, Lin HM, Hulstyn MJ, et al. Lateral meniscus root tear and meniscus extrusion with anterior cruciate ligament tear. Radiology 2006;239(3):805–10.

[25] Hunter DJ, Zhang YQ, Niu JB, et al. The association of meniscal pathologic changes with cartilage loss in symptomatic knee osteoarthritis. Arthritis Rheum 2006;54(3):795–801.

[26] Hough AJ Jr, Webber RJ. Pathology of the meniscus. Clin Orthop Relat Res Mar 1990;(252):32–40.

[27] Vedi V, Williams A, Tennant SJ, et al. Meniscal movement. An in-vivo study using dynamic MRI. J Bone Joint Surg Br 1999;81(1):37–41.

[28] Jee WH, McCauley TR, Kim JM, et al. Meniscal tear configurations: categorization with MR imaging. AJR Am J Roentgenol 2003;180(1):93–7.

[29] De Smet AA, Norris MA, Yandow DR, et al. MR diagnosis of meniscal tears of the knee: importance of high signal in the meniscus that extends to the surface. AJR Am J Roentgenol 1993;161(1):101–7.

[30] Drosos GI, Pozo JL. The causes and mechanisms of meniscal injuries in the sporting and non-sporting environment in an unselected population. Knee 2004;11(2):143–9.

[31] Escobedo EM, Hunter JC, Zink-Brody GC, et al. Usefulness of turbo spin-echo MR imaging in the evaluation of meniscal tears: comparison with a conventional spin-echo sequence. AJR Am J Roentgenol 1996;167(5):1223–7.

[32] Helms CA. The meniscus: recent advances in MR imaging of the knee. AJR Am J Roentgenol 2002;179(5):1115–22.

[33] Oei EH, Nikken JJ, Verstijnen AC, et al. MR imaging of the menisci and cruciate ligaments: a systematic review. Radiology 2003;226(3):837–48.

[34] De Smet AA, Norris MA, Yandow DR, et al. Diagnosis of meniscal tears of the knee with MR imaging: effect of observer variation and sample size on sensitivity and specificity. AJR Am J Roentgenol 1993;160(3):555–9.

[35] De Smet AA, Tuite MJ. Use of the "two-slice-touch" rule for the MRI diagnosis of meniscal tears. AJR Am J Roentgenol 2006;187(4):911–4.

[36] Rubin DA, Kneeland JB, Listerud J, et al. MR diagnosis of meniscal tears of the knee: value of fast spin-echo vs conventional spin-echo pulse sequences. AJR Am J Roentgenol 1994;162(5):1131–5.

[37] Kowalchuk RM, Kneeland JB, Dalinka MK, et al. MRI of the knee: value of short echo time fast spin-echo using high performance gradients versus conventional spin-echo imaging for the detection of meniscal tears. Skeletal Radiol 2000;29(9):520–4.

[38] Chang CY, Wu HT, Huang TF, et al. Imaging evaluation of meniscal injury of the knee joint: a comparative MR imaging and arthroscopic study. Clin Imaging 2004;28(5):372–6.

[39] Guckel C, Jundt G, Schnabel K, et al. Spin-echo and 3D gradient-echo imaging of the knee joint: a clinical and histopathological comparison. Eur J Radiol 1995;21(1):25–33.

[40] Cheung LP, Li KC, Hollett MD, et al. Meniscal tears of the knee: accuracy of detection with fast spin-echo MR imaging and arthroscopic correlation in 293 patients. Radiology 1997;203(2):508–12.

[41] Vande Berg BC, Malghem J, Poilvache P, et al. Meniscal tears with fragments displaced in notch and recesses of knee: MR imaging with arthroscopic comparison. Radiology 2005;234(3):842–50.

[42] Blackmon GB, Major NM, Helms CA. Comparison of fast spin-echo versus conventional spin-echo MRI for evaluating meniscal tears. AJR Am J Roentgenol 2005;184(6):1740–3.

[43] Heron CW, Calvert PT. Three-dimensional gradient-echo MR imaging of the knee: comparison with arthroscopy in 100 patients. Radiology 1992;183(3):839–44.

[44] Reeder JD, Matz SO, Becker L, et al. MR imaging of the knee in the sagittal projection: comparison of three-dimensional gradient-echo and spin-echo sequences. AJR Am J Roentgenol 1989;153(3):537–40.

[45] Hodler J, Haghighi P, Pathria MN, et al. Meniscal changes in the elderly: correlation of MR imaging and histologic findings. Radiology 1992;184(1):221–5.

[46] Magee T, Williams D. Detection of meniscal tears and marrow lesions using coronal MRI. AJR Am J Roentgenol 2004;183(5):1469–73.

[47] Magee TH, Hinson GW. MRI of meniscal bucket-handle tears. Skeletal Radiol 1998;27(9):495–9.

[48] Tarhan NC, Chung CB, Mohana-Borges AV, et al. Meniscal tears: role of axial MRI alone and in combination with other imaging planes. AJR Am J Roentgenol 2004;183(1):9–15.

[49] Lee JH, Singh TT, Bolton G. Axial fat-saturated FSE imaging of knee: appearance of meniscal tears. Skeletal Radiol 2002;31(7):384–95.

[50] White LM, Schweitzer ME, Weishaupt D, et al. Diagnosis of recurrent meniscal tears: prospective evaluation of conventional MR imaging, indirect MR arthrography, and direct MR arthrography. Radiology 2002;222(2):421–9.

[51] Deutsch AL, Mink JH, Fox JM, et al. Peripheral meniscal tears: MR findings after conservative treatment or arthroscopic repair. Radiology 1990;176(2):485–8.

[52] Quinn SF, Brown TF. Meniscal tears diagnosed with MR imaging versus arthroscopy: how reliable a standard is arthroscopy? Radiology 1991; 181(3):843–7.

[53] Boxheimer L, Lutz AM, Zanetti M, et al. Characteristics of displaceable and nondisplaceable meniscal tears at kinematic MR imaging of the knee. Radiology 2006;238(1):221–31.

[54] Magee T, Shapiro M, Williams D. MR accuracy and arthroscopic incidence of meniscal radial tears. Skeletal Radiol 2002;31(12):686–9.

[55] Tuckman GA, Miller WJ, Remo JW, et al. Radial tears of the menisci: MR findings. AJR Am J Roentgenol 1994;163(2):395–400.

[56] Kidron A, Thein R. Radial tears associated with cleavage tears of the medial meniscus in athletes. Arthroscopy 2002;18(3):254–6.

[57] Ruff C, Weingardt JP, Russ PD, et al. MR imaging patterns of displaced meniscus injuries of the knee. AJR Am J Roentgenol 1998;170(1):63–7.

[58] Lecas LK, Helms CA, Kosarek FJ, et al. Inferiorly displaced flap tears of the medial meniscus: MR appearance and clinical significance. AJR Am J Roentgenol 2000;174(1):161–4.

[59] Watt AJ, Halliday T, Raby N. The value of the absent bow tie sign in MRI of bucket-handle tears. Clin Radiol 2000;55(8):622–6.

[60] Ververidis AN, Verettas DA, Kazakos KJ, et al. Meniscal bucket handle tears: a retrospective study of arthroscopy and the relation to MRI. Knee Surg Sports Traumatol Arthrosc 2006; 14(4):343–9.

[61] Dorsay TA, Helms CA. Bucket-handle meniscal tears of the knee: sensitivity and specificity of MRI signs. Skeletal Radiol 2003;32(5):266–72.

[62] Wright DH, De Smet AA, Norris M. Bucket-handle tears of the medial and lateral menisci of the knee: value of MR imaging in detecting displaced fragments. AJR Am J Roentgenol 1995; 165(3):621–5.

[63] Aydingoz U, Firat AK, Atay OA, et al. MR imaging of meniscal bucket-handle tears: a review of signs and their relation to arthroscopic classification. Eur Radiol 2003;13(3):618–25.

[64] Helms CA, Laorr A, Cannon WD Jr. The absent bow tie sign in bucket-handle tears of the menisci in the knee. AJR Am J Roentgenol 1998;170(1):57–61.

[65] Singson RD, Feldman F, Staron R, et al. MR imaging of displaced bucket-handle tear of the medial meniscus. AJR Am J Roentgenol 1991; 156(1):121–4.

[66] Weiss KL, Morehouse HT, Levy IM. Sagittal MR images of the knee: a low-signal band parallel to the posterior cruciate ligament caused by a displaced bucket-handle tear. AJR Am J Roentgenol 1991;156(1):117–9.

[67] Bugnone AN, Ramnath RR, Davis SB, et al. The quadruple cruciate sign of simultaneous bicompartmental medial and lateral bucket-handle meniscal tears. Skeletal Radiol 2005;34(11): 740–4.

[68] Jee WH, McCauley TR, Kim JM. Magnetic resonance diagnosis of meniscal tears in patients with acute anterior cruciate ligament tears. J Comput Assist Tomogr 2004;28(3):402–6.

[69] De Smet AA, Graf BK. Meniscal tears missed on MR imaging: relationship to meniscal tear patterns and anterior cruciate ligament tears. AJR Am J Roentgenol 1994;162(4):905–11.

[70] von Eisenhart-Rothe R, Bringmann C, Siebert M, et al. Femoro-tibial and meniscotibial translation patterns in patients with unilateral anterior cruciate ligament deficiency—a potential cause of secondary meniscal tears. J Orthop Res 2004;22(2):275–82.

[71] Mink JH, Levy T, Crues JV 3rd. Tears of the anterior cruciate ligament and menisci of the knee: MR imaging evaluation. Radiology 1988; 167(3):769–74.

[72] Sproule JA, Khan F, Rice JJ, et al. Altered signal intensity in the posterior horn of the medial meniscus: an MR finding of questionable significance. Arch Orthop Trauma Surg 2005;125(4):267–71.

[73] Peterfy CG, Janzen DL, Tirman PF, et al. "Magic-angle" phenomenon: a cause of increased signal in the normal lateral meniscus on short-TE MR images of the knee. AJR Am J Roentgenol 1994; 163(1):149–54.

[74] Turner DA, Rapoport MI, Erwin WD, et al. Truncation artifact: a potential pitfall in MR imaging of the menisci of the knee. Radiology 1991;179(3):629–33.

[75] Shankman S, Beltran J, Melamed E, et al. Anterior horn of the lateral meniscus: another potential pitfall in MR imaging of the knee. Radiology 1997;204(1):181–4.

[76] Herman LJ, Beltran J. Pitfalls in MR imaging of the knee. Radiology 1988;167(3):775–81.

[77] Vahey TN, Bennett HT, Arrington LE, et al. MR imaging of the knee: pseudotear of the lateral meniscus caused by the meniscofemoral ligament. AJR Am J Roentgenol 1990;154(6):1237–9.

[78] Sanders TG, Linares RC, Lawhorn KW, et al. Oblique meniscomeniscal ligament: another potential pitfall for a meniscal tear—anatomic description and appearance at MR imaging in three cases. Radiology 1999;213(1):213–6.

[79] Soejima T, Murakami H, Tanaka N, et al. Anteromedial meniscofemoral ligament. Arthroscopy 2003;19(1):90–5.

[80] Cothran RL Jr, Major NM, Helms CA, et al. MR imaging of meniscal contusion in the knee. AJR Am J Roentgenol 2001;177(5):1189–92.

[81] Kaushik S, Erickson JK, Palmer WE, et al. Effect of chondrocalcinosis on the MR imaging of knee menisci. AJR Am J Roentgenol 2001; 177(4):905–9.

[82] Rubin DA, Britton CA, Towers JD, et al. Are MR imaging signs of meniscocapsular separation valid? Radiology 1996;201(3):829–36.

[83] De Maeseneer M, Lenchik L, Starok M, et al. Normal and abnormal medial meniscocapsular structures: MR imaging and sonography in cadavers. AJR Am J Roentgenol 1998;171(4): 969–76.

[84] De Maeseneer M, Shahabpour M, Vanderdood K, et al. Medial meniscocapsular separation: MR imaging criteria and diagnostic pitfalls. Eur J Radiol 2002;41(3):242–52.

[85] De Smet AA, Asinger DA, Johnson RL. Abnormal superior popliteomeniscal fascicle and posterior pericapsular edema: indirect MR imaging signs of a lateral meniscal tear. AJR Am J Roentgenol 2001;176(1):63–6.

[86] Blankenbaker DG, De Smet AA, Smith JD. Usefulness of two indirect MR imaging signs to diagnose lateral meniscal tears. AJR Am J Roentgenol 2002;178(3):579–82.

[87] Yao L, Stanczak J, Boutin RD. Presumptive subarticular stress reactions of the knee: MRI detection and association with meniscal tear patterns. Skeletal Radiol 2004;33(5): 260–4.

[88] Muscolo DL, Costa-Paz M, Ayerza M, et al. Medial meniscal tears and spontaneous osteonecrosis of the knee. Arthroscopy 2006;22(4): 457–60.

[89] Brahme SK, Fox JM, Ferkel RD, et al. Osteonecrosis of the knee after arthroscopic surgery: diagnosis with MR imaging. Radiology 1991; 178(3):851–3.

[90] Kaplan PA, Gehl RH, Dussault RG, et al. Bone contusions of the posterior lip of the medial tibial plateau (contrecoup injury) and associated internal derangements of the knee at MR imaging. Radiology 1999;211(3): 747–53.

[91] Campbell SE, Sanders TG, Morrison WB. MR imaging of meniscal cysts: incidence, location, and clinical significance. AJR Am J Roentgenol 2001;177(2):409–13.

[92] De Maeseneer M, Shahabpour M, Vanderdood K, et al. MR imaging of meniscal cysts: evaluation of location and extension using a three-layer approach. Eur J Radiol 2001;39(2):117–24.

[93] Lektrakul N, Skaf A, Yeh L, et al. Pericruciate meniscal cysts arising from tears of the posterior horn of the medial meniscus: MR imaging features that simulate posterior cruciate

ganglion cysts. AJR Am J Roentgenol 1999; 172(6):1575–9.

[94] Riel KA, Reinisch M, Kersting-Sommerhoff B, et al. 0.2-Tesla magnetic resonance imaging of internal lesions of the knee joint: a prospective arthroscopically controlled clinical study. Knee Surg Sports Traumatol Arthrosc 1999;7(1): 37–41.

[95] Cotten A, Delfaut E, Demondion X, et al. MR imaging of the knee at 0.2 and 1.5 T: correlation with surgery. AJR Am J Roentgenol 2000; 174(4):1093–7.

[96] Rand T, Imhof H, Turetschek K, et al. Comparison of low field (0.2T) and high field (1.5T) MR imaging in the differentiation of torned from intact menisci. Eur J Radiol 1999;30(1):22–7.

[97] Toms AP, White LM, Marshall TJ, et al. Imaging the post-operative meniscus. Eur J Radiol 2005; 54(2):189–98.

[98] Steenbrugge F, Verdonk R, Verstraete K. Long-term assessment of arthroscopic meniscus repair: a 13-year follow-up study. Knee 2002; 9(3):181–7.

[99] Pena E, Calvo B, Martinez MA, et al. Finite element analysis of the effect of meniscal tears and meniscectomies on human knee biomechanics. Clin Biomech (Bristol, Avon) 2005;20(5): 498–507.

[100] Farley TE, Howell SM, Love KF, et al. Meniscal tears: MR and arthrographic findings after arthroscopic repair. Radiology 1991;180(2):517–22.

[101] Magee T, Shapiro M, Williams D. Prevalence of meniscal radial tears of the knee revealed by MRI after surgery. AJR Am J Roentgenol 2004; 182(4):931–6.

[102] White LM, Kramer J, Recht MP. MR imaging evaluation of the postoperative knee: ligaments, menisci, and articular cartilage. Skeletal Radiol 2005;34(8):431–52.

[103] Zanetti M, Pfirrmann CW, Schmid MR, et al. Patients with suspected meniscal tears: prevalence of abnormalities seen on MRI of 100 symptomatic and 100 contralateral asymptomatic knees. AJR Am J Roentgenol 2003;181(3):635–41.

[104] Potter HG, Rodeo SA, Wickiewicz TL, et al. MR imaging of meniscal allografts: correlation with clinical and arthroscopic outcomes. Radiology 1996;198(2):509–14.

[105] Sgaglione NA, Steadman JR, Shaffer B, et al. Current concepts in meniscus surgery: resection to replacement. Arthroscopy 2003;19(Suppl 1): 161–88.

[106] Donahue TL, Hull ML, Howell SM. New algorithm for selecting meniscal allografts that best match the size and shape of the damaged meniscus. J Orthop Res 2006;24(7):1535–43.

[107] Shaffer B, Kennedy S, Klimkiewicz J, et al. Preoperative sizing of meniscal allografts in meniscus transplantation. Am J Sports Med 2000; 28(4):524–33.

[108] Sciulli RL, Boutin RD, Brown RR, et al. Evaluation of the postoperative meniscus of the knee:

a study comparing conventional arthrography, conventional MR imaging, MR arthrography with iodinated contrast material, and MR arthrography with gadolinium-based contrast material. Skeletal Radiol 1999;28(9):508–14.

[109] Hantes ME, Zachos VC, Zibis AH, et al. Evaluation of meniscal repair with serial magnetic resonance imaging: a comparative study between conventional MRI and indirect MR arthrography. Eur J Radiol 2004;50(3):231–7.

[110] Applegate GR, Flannigan BD, Tolin BS, et al. MR diagnosis of recurrent tears in the knee: value of intraarticular contrast material. AJR Am J Roentgenol 1993;161(4):821–5.

[111] Vives MJ, Homesley D, Ciccotti MG, et al. Evaluation of recurring meniscal tears with gadolinium-enhanced magnetic resonance imaging: a randomized, prospective study. Am J Sports Med 2003;31(6):868–73.

[112] Magee T, Shapiro M, Rodriguez J, et al. MR arthrography of postoperative knee: for which patients is it useful? Radiology 2003;229(1):159–63.

[113] Smith DK, Totty WG. The knee after partial meniscectomy: MR imaging features. Radiology 1990;176(1):141–4.

[114] Verdonk PC, Verstraete KL, Almqvist KF, et al. Meniscal allograft transplantation: long-term clinical results with radiological and magnetic resonance imaging correlations. Knee Surg Sports Traumatol Arthrosc 2006;14(8):694–706.

[115] van Arkel ER, Goei R, de Ploeg I, et al. Meniscal allografts: evaluation with magnetic resonance imaging and correlation with arthroscopy. Arthroscopy 2000;16(5):517–21.

[116] Patten RM, Rolfe BA. MRI of meniscal allografts. J Comput Assist Tomogr 1995;19(2):243–6.

[117] Verdonk P, Depaepe Y, Desmyter S, et al. Normal and transplanted lateral knee menisci: evaluation of extrusion using magnetic resonance imaging and ultrasound. Knee Surg Sports Traumatol Arthrosc 2004;12(5):411–9.

[118] Gatehouse PD, Thomas RW, Robson MD, et al. Magnetic resonance imaging of the knee with ultrashort TE pulse sequences. Magn Reson Imaging 2004;22(8):1061–7.

[119] Gatehouse PD, He T, Puri BK, et al. Contrast-enhanced MRI of the menisci of the knee using ultrashort echo time (UTE) pulse sequences: imaging of the red and white zones. Br J Radiol 2004;77(920):641–7.

[120] Kreitner KF, Romaneehsen B, Krummenauer F, et al. Fast magnetic resonance imaging of the knee using a parallel acquisition technique (mSENSE): a prospective performance evaluation. Eur Radiol 2006;16(8):1659–66.

[121] Niitsu M, Ikeda K. Routine MR examination of the knee using parallel imaging. Clin Radiol 2003;58(10):801–7.

[122] Ramnath RR, Magee T, Wasudev N, et al. Accuracy of 3-T MRI using fast spin-echo technique to detect meniscal tears of the knee. AJR Am J Roentgenol 2006;187(1):221–5.

[123] Magee T, Williams D. 3.0-T MRI of meniscal tears. AJR Am J Roentgenol 2006;187(2):371–5.

[124] Craig JG, Go L, Blechinger J, et al. Three-tesla imaging of the knee: initial experience. Skeletal Radiol 2005;34(8):453–61.

RADIOLOGIC
CLINICS
OF NORTH AMERICA

Radiol Clin N Am 45 (2007) 1055–1062

ELSEVIER
SAUNDERS

Three-Tesla MR Imaging of the Knee

Thomas Magee, MD

- MR protocols
- Artifacts
  - *Specific absorption rate*
  - *Susceptibility artifact*
  - *Chemical shift artifacts*
- Clinical utility of 3-Tesla imaging
- Future developments
- Summary
- References

MR imaging has been found to be highly accurate in the diagnosis of knee pathology. In previous studies, the sensitivity of MR imaging in the detection of meniscal tears has been reported to be between 80% and 100% [1–7]. MR accuracy in detection of anterior cruciate ligament, posterior cruciate ligament, and collateral ligament injuries has also been reported to be highly accurate [1–7].

Three-tesla (3-T) MR imaging has been available since 2001 [8]. Since that time, 3-T imaging has grown to be an important part of the overall imaging market. The higher signal/noise ratio (SNR) afforded by 3-T imaging allows for better image quality leading to higher diagnostic accuracy. The high SNR can increase imaging speed and/or spatial resolution. One can also enhance SNR, spatial resolution, and contrast/noise ratio to allow more accurate diagnosis of pathologic conditions with use of a 3-T system.

The author's practice has used 3-T MR imaging since 2003, exclusively for knee imaging. They have adjusted the imaging parameters slightly from those they performed on their 1.5-T MR to optimize high-resolution imaging on their 3-T system. These high-resolution images have resulted in an increased accuracy in their diagnoses as well as faster throughput of patients.

MR protocols

MR imaging of the knee with 3-T (as with any field strength) should include sequences in all three planes, including coronal, axial, and sagittal images. In the author's practice, a 3-T GE Signa scanner (General Electric Medical Systems, Milwaukee, Wisconsin) is used, although there are various 3-T platforms offered by several manufacturers. The author's practice uses coronal fast spin-echo T1-weighted (750/10, echo time/repetition time [TR/TE]) coronal, sagittal, and axial fast spin-echo fat saturated T2-weighted (3950/51, TR/TE), and fast spin-echo proton density sagittal (1800/12, TR/TE) sequences with a field of view of 15 cm on all images. Slice thickness is 3 mm with a 10% interslice gap on all sequences except for the fast spin-echo proton density sagittal sequence, which has a 2-mm slice thickness with a 10% interslice gap. The matrix on the sagittal proton density sequence is 416 × 288, whereas the matrix on all other sequences is 320 × 320. The echo train lengths are 3 for the T1 coronal, 6 for the fast spin-echo sagittal proton density sequence, and 12 for all other sequences. Two number of excitations (NEX) are used on all sequences apart from the T1 coronal sequence in which one NEX is used. The author's practice uses a quadrature extremity coil for

This article was originally published in *Magnetic Resonance Imaging Clinics of North America* 15:1, February 2007.
Neuroskeletal Imaging, 1344 Apollo Boulevard, Suite 406, Melbourne, FL 32901, USA
E-mail address: tmageerad@cfl.rr.com

imaging of the knee; however several other coils are also available.

Artifacts

MR imaging parameters at 3-T must be modified from those at 1.5-T because of potential artifacts that may be more pronounced than on 1.5-T MR units. Specific issues to be addressed at 3-T include specific absorption rate (SAR), chemical shift artifact, susceptibility artifacts, T1 time prolongation, and T2 time shortening.

Three-tesla MR imaging allows for a higher SNR compared with 1.5-T MR imaging. The spin–spin relaxation time, T2, remains fairly constant at different field strengths. However, the spin–lattice relaxation time, T1, increases as the field strength increases. Therefore, at 3-T, the TR must be longer than on 1.5-T MR scanners to maximize the SNR gain. At 3-T, the TR must be longer to attain the same type of contrast on T1-weighted images as seen on a 1.5-T scanner. Also on 3-T MR scanners, the TE must be slightly shorter than on 1.5-T MR scanners to account for decreased T2 relaxation time [9,10].

The parameters the author's practice uses for imaging of the knee at 3-T have an increased TR and a decreased TE on all sequences compared with parameters previously used on their 1.5-T MR scanners. This was done to optimize SNR on the 3-T MR.

Three-tesla imaging allows for a higher SNR compared with 1.5-T imaging. This can be used to improve imaging speed or resolution. However, there is increased T1 relaxation time and decreased T2 relaxation time at 3-T compared with 1.5-T. Also at 3-T, there is increased sensitivity to magnetic susceptibility artifacts and chemical shift artifacts as compared with 1.5-T. To reduce the chemical shift artifact, the author's practice doubled their bandwidth with 3-T compared with their bandwidth used at 1.5-T. Doubling the bandwidth results in a reduction of SNR by the square root of 2. The increase in SNR afforded at higher field strength has allowed for faster imaging at 3-T with improved resolution and thinner slice thickness compared with 1.5-T [10]. In the author's practice, they have experienced faster throughput, higher resolution imaging, and they feel more confident in making a diagnosis of a meniscal tear after changing to 3-T imaging from 1.5-T imaging.

Specific absorption rate

SAR describes the energy deposited in a patient. SAR increases with the magnetic field strength. The SAR deposited in a tissue is proportional to the duty cycle and the amount of tissue being scanned. SAR is exponentially proportional to the magnetic field strength and flip angle. SAR is increased by high duty cycles (shorter TRs and more radiofrequency pulses) as with fast spin-echo techniques. SAR effects are more severe with fast spin-echo than with spin-echo, and least severe with gradient echo sequences. Larger body parts are subject to more SAR [8].

One way to decrease SAR is to increase the TR value for a given sequence. This decreases the duty cycle by increasing the cooling time between repetition pulses. Doubling the TR decreases the SNR by 2 [8]. Use of transmit–receive surface coils or extremity coils also markedly reduce the amount of body tissue exposed to radiofrequency waves thereby reducing SAR.

Parallel imaging (as used with phased array coils) also reduces the duty cycle thereby decreasing SAR [8]. Parallel imaging uses spatial data derived from phased-array coil elements to construct a portion of k-space. Fewer echoes than traditional techniques are used to obtain desired resolution. MR spatial information is traditionally acquired through the application of rapidly switching magnetic gradients and radiofrequency pulses. Most of the fast imaging techniques achieve high speeds by optimizing switching rates and patterns of gradients and pulses. However, these techniques acquire data in a sequential fashion. Thus, imaging speed is limited by the maximum switching rates. Higher switching rates increase the duty cycle, which in turn increases SAR. Parallel imaging allows encoding of multiple lines of MR data simultaneously. This has resulted in a twofold to fivefold increase in acquisition speed in vivo. Parallel imaging results in a reduction of scan time, better spatial resolution in a given imaging time, and less degradation of image quality due to motion. Parallel imaging results in a decreased scan time and a decrease in SAR. However, parallel imaging also results in a decrease in overall SNR. The author's practice uses a parallel imaging capable eight-channel phased array knee coil [8] and have been able to produce high-resolution images more quickly. An entire knee MR examination can be completed in less than 5 minutes with use of parallel imaging (Figs. 1–3).

Susceptibility artifact

Metallic hardware produces susceptibility artifact. This is more pronounced at higher field strengths. Lengthening the echo train length decreases susceptibility but results in increased SAR. Increasing bandwidth decreases the susceptibility artifact but results in a decrease SNR. Short tau inversion recovery sequences can be used instead of chemically selective fat saturated T2-weighted sequences to decrease susceptibility artifact [8]. Parallel imaging also decreases susceptibility artifact (Figs. 4 and 5).

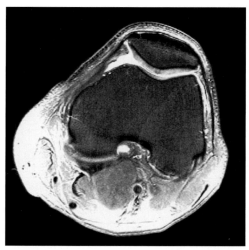

Fig. 1. High-resolution axial intermediate weighted image with fat saturation (TR/TE 3950/51) MR image of the knee produced with parallel imaging.

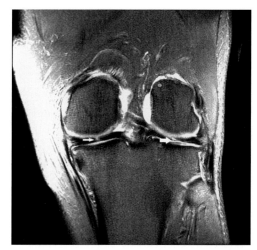

Fig. 3. High-resolution coronal intermediate weighted image with fat saturation (TR/TE 3950/51) MR image of the knee produced with parallel imaging.

Chemical shift artifacts

Chemical shift artifacts are more pronounced at 3-T than at other field strengths. Chemical shift artifact at 3-T is twice that of 1.5-T. This artifact occurs because with frequency encoding, fat protons precess slower than water protons in the same slice. Due to this difference in resonance frequency between water and fat, protons at the same location become misregistered (displaced) by the fourier transformation, when converting MR imaging signal from frequency to spatial domain. This chemical shift misregistration causes accentuation of any fat–water interfaces along the frequency axis and may be mistaken for pathology. At any fat–water interface, this artifact can be seen as a bright or dark band at the edge of the anatomy. This artifact is more pronounced at higher field strengths [9,10]. In the author's practice, they double the bandwidth (which results in decreased SNR) to decrease the chemical shift artifact on 3-T scanners (Figs. 6–8) [10].

Clinical utility of 3-Tesla imaging

Three-tesla MR imaging of the knee is sensitive and specific for detection of meniscal tears when compared with arthroscopy. Previous studies have demonstrated MR imaging at 1.5-T field strength or less

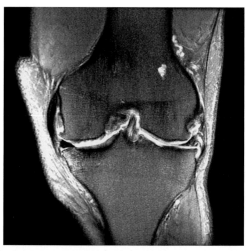

Fig. 2. High-resolution coronal intermediate weighted image with fat saturation (TR/TE 3950/51) MR image of the knee produced with parallel imaging.

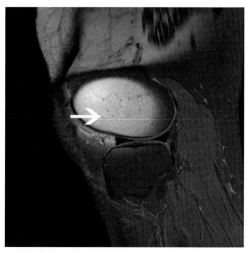

Fig. 4. Sagittal fat saturated intermediate weighted image (TR/TE 3950/51) MR knee demonstrates considerable blooming artifact (*arrow*).

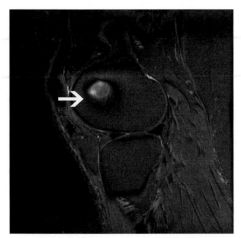

Fig. 5. Sagittal short tau inversion recovery MR knee in the same patient demonstrates considerably less blooming artifact (*arrow*).

to be sensitive for detection of meniscal tears [1–6]. The author's practice uses 3-T MR imaging exclusively for imaging the knee, because they feel more confident in making a diagnosis of a meniscal tear with 3-T imaging when compared with 1.5-T imaging. Some authors have advocated equivocating on the diagnosis of a meniscal tear in up to 10% of cases when using a 1.5-T MR [11]. Anecdotally, the author seldom if ever feels a need to equivocate as to whether a meniscal tear is present with 3-T imaging and therefore feels that knee MR imaging at 3-T allows for more accurate and definitive diagnoses compared with imaging at 1.5-T.

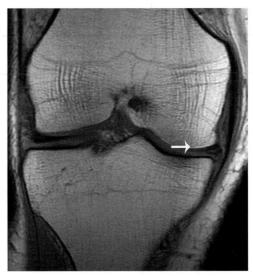

Fig. 7. Moderate bandwidth of 41.67 kHz results in moderate chemical shift artifact at articular surface (*arrow*).

The parameters used with MR imaging of the knee with 3-T have increased TR and decreased TE on all sequences compared with parameters used on 1.5-T MR. This is done to optimize SNR with 3-T MR. Three-tesla imaging allows for a higher SNR as compared with 1.5-T imaging. However there is increased T1 relaxation time and decreased T2 relaxation time at 3-T compared with 1.5-T. Also at 3-T, there is increased sensitivity to magnetic susceptibility artifacts and chemical shift artifacts compared with 1.5-T. To reduce the chemical shift artifact, the author's practice doubles their

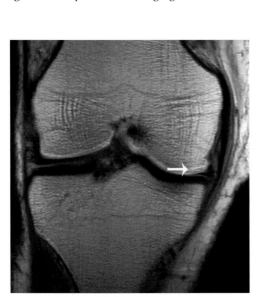

Fig. 6. Low bandwidth of 10.42 kHz results in considerable chemical shift artifact at articular surface (*arrow*).

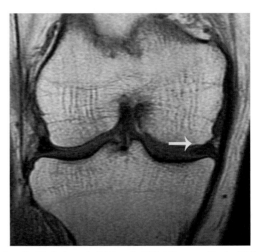

Fig. 8. High bandwidth of 100 kHz results in little chemical shift artifact at articular surface (*arrow*).

A B

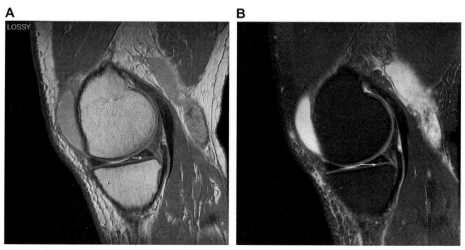

Fig. 9. (A, B) Subtle meniscal tear demonstrated at 3-T with sagittal intermediate weighted image (TR/TE 1800/12) (arrow).

bandwidth on 3-T compared with bandwidth used at 1.5-T. The increase in SNR allows for faster imaging at 3-T with improved resolution and thinner slice thickness compared with 1.5-T [10].

The author's practice routinely correlates MR interpretations with arthroscopy as a part of a quality-assurance program. As an offshoot of that quality assessment program, two studies were recently published relating to the accuracy of 3-T MR imaging for the detection of meniscal tears. In one study, MR sensitivity for detection of meniscal tears with 3-T imaging of the knee was 96%, with 108 out of 112 meniscal tears seen at arthroscopy were detected with MR imaging (95% confidence interval, 92.8%–98.2%). Specificity was 97%

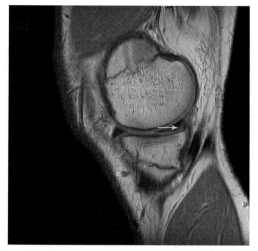

Fig. 10. Subtle meniscal tear demonstrated at 3-T (arrow).

(95% confidence interval, 93%–98.3%) [12]. In the other study by Ramnath and colleagues [13], MR sensitivity for detection of meniscal tears was 95% and the specificity was 92%. In both studies, subtle meniscal tears were accurately diagnosed with 3-T imaging. Both studies logically concluded that if a meniscal tear was not seen on a 3-T MR examination, there was little likelihood of finding a tear at arthroscopy. This accuracy aids surgeons in determining patients who need surgical intervention versus those who would benefit from rehabilitation and physical therapy (Figs. 9 and 10).

Both authors found fast spin-echo imaging at 3-T to be highly accurate in the diagnosis of meniscal tears. A high echo train length used in fast spin-echo imaging could theoretically worsen spatial blurring because of the contribution of lower signals to the edges of k-space. In practice however, this did not affect the author's ability to diagnose meniscal tears. This may be because of the high in-plane spatial resolution and the decreased slice thickness used in sagittal fast spin-echo nonfat saturated proton density sequence. The added signal to noise ratio with 3-T systems likely compensates for the diminished signal in the outer lines of k-space on fast spin-echo sequences and reduces the degree of blurring [12,13].

A previous study indicated that signal should touch a surface on two images to definitively report a meniscal tear on MR [6]. In the author's studies, if signal was definitively seen to touch a surface on one view, a meniscal tear was reported. Using the criteria in the author's study did not decrease specificity (97%) compared with previous studies performed on 1.5-T or lower field strength. This may be due to the high-resolution images afforded by

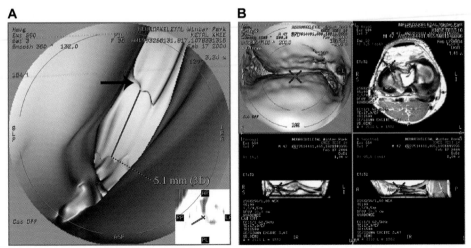

Fig. 11. (A) Three-dimensional rendering of meniscal tear (*arrow*) obtained with 3-T MR imaging on virtual arthroscopy. (B) Three-dimensional rendering of knee to produce movie clip for virtual arthroscopy. The knee is also visualized in coronal, axial, and sagittal planes for accurate visualization of location on three-dimensional movie rendering.

3-T imaging. Alternately this may be due to thin-section (2 mm) proton density sagittal images. In previous studies, slice thickness on sagittal proton density images was at least 3 mm. The thinner sections may make it clearer to determine whether or not signal touches the surface of the meniscus. In the author's previous study, six cases demonstrated signal to touch a meniscal surface on one view only. In all six cases, a meniscal tear was seen at arthroscopy [12]. Four of these were meniscal radial tears (which often are only seen on one view), whereas two were horizontal tears seen to touch a surface on only a single image [12].

Future developments

Recent innovations in technology allow near isotropic imaging of the knee at 3-T with proton density meniscal imaging able to be obtained in 6 minutes or less. Images can be acquired in the axial plane (at 0.3-mm slice thickness) and reconstructed in the sagittal and coronal planes. The reconstructed images provide the same clinical information that the de novo images provide. Additionally three-dimensional images and movie clips can be produced, which can provide the surgeon with "virtual arthroscopy." This allows the surgeon to have more

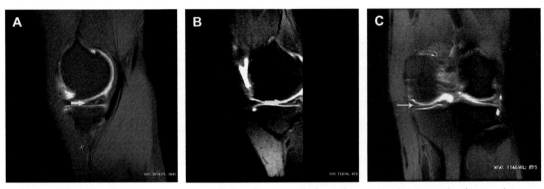

Fig. 12. (A) MR arthrogram of the knee acquired in the sagittal plane demonstrating a meniscal retear in a post-operative knee (*arrow*). (B) MR arthrographic image demonstrates meniscal retear on sagittal reconstructed image derived from near-isotropic images acquired in the axial plane (*arrow*). (C) MR arthrographic image demonstrates meniscal retear on coronal reconstructed image derived from near-isotropic images acquired in the axial plane (*arrow*).

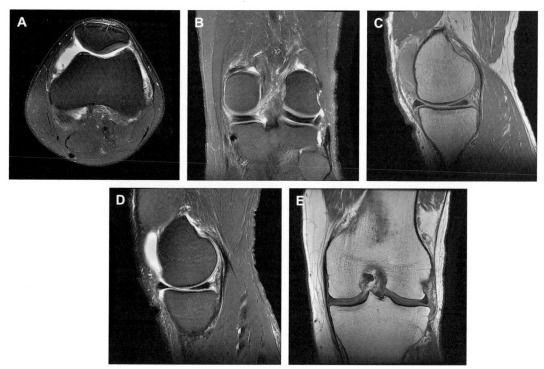

Fig. 13. (*A*) Axial fat saturated intermediate weighted image of the knee (TR/TE 3950/51). (*B*) Coronal fat saturated intermediate weighted image of the knee (TR/TE 3950/51). (*C*) Sagittal intermediate weighted image of the knee (TR/TE 1800/12). (*D*) Sagittal fat saturated intermediate weighted image of the knee (TR/TE 3950/51). (*E*) Coronal T1-weighted image of the knee (TR/TE 750/10).

exact information regarding the location and degree of displacement (if any) of the meniscal tears and facilitates presurgical planning (Figs. 11A, B and 12A–C).

Parallel imaging allows for fast high-resolution imaging of the knee. With the use of an eight-channel phased array knee coil, one can produce an entire knee examination in less than 5 minutes with high-resolution images (see Figs. 1–3). Continuous improvements in coil technology now allow superb high-resolution images to be produced with conventional imaging using an eight-channel knee coil (Fig. 13A–E). Continued future coil development will allow for even higher resolution imaging at 3-T.

Three-tesla MR imaging likely benefits articular cartilage imaging in addition to evaluating meniscal pathology. Early studies with 3-T imaging have indicated that higher field strength provides greater diagnostic accuracy in detection of focal chondral defects [14]. Studies have indicated improved contrast to noise of the cartilage/bone and cartilage/fluid interface at 3-T compared with 1.5-T [14]. Three-tesla imaging is also proving useful for T2 cartilage mapping, which can help with respect to demonstration of early degenerative changes of

articular cartilage before they become evident on an anatomic basis [14]. Early studies at 3-T have also indicated a greater diagnostic accuracy of 3-T in detection of articular hyaline cartilage defects [14], and more thorough evaluations are likely to follow in the near future.

Summary

Three-tesla MR imaging of the knee allows for fast, accurate high-resolution imaging. Studies have found 3-T MR imaging to be highly accurate in detection of meniscal tears, which is clinically useful for treatment planning [12,13]. It has been shown that if a meniscal tear is not seen on 3-T MR imaging, it is highly unlikely to be present. Three-dimensional imaging of the knee is also being developed and evaluated, and referring physicians have found virtual arthroscopy to be beneficial for presurgical planning. Early data also depict 3-T MR to be highly accurate in assessment of articular cartilage defects, and T2 cartilage mapping can be more easily performed on 3-T MR. This may also help in diagnosis and treatment of osteoarthritic changes about the knee before they become anatomically evident.

References

[1] Kelly MA, Flock TJ, Kimmel JA, et al. MR Imaging of the knee: clarification of its role. Arthroscopy 1991;7:78–85.

[2] Mink JH, Deutsch AL, Crues JV, et al. MR imaging of the knee: technical factors, diagnostic accuracy, and further pitfalls. Radiology 1987; 165:175–9.

[3] Crues JV, Mink J, Levy TL, et al. Meniscal tears of the knee: accuracy of MR imaging. Radiology 1987;164:445–8.

[4] DeSmet AA, Norris MA, Yandow DR, et al. Diagnosis of meniscal tears of the knee with MR imaging: effect of observer variation and sample size on sensitivity and specificity. AJR Am J Roentgenol 1993;160:555–9.

[5] DeSmet AA, Tuite MJ, Norris MA, et al. MR diagnosis of meniscal tears: analysis of causes of errors. AJR Am J Roentgenol 1994;163: 1419–23.

[6] DeSmet AA, Norris MA, Yandow DR, et al. MR diagnosis of meniscal tears of the knee: importance of high signal in the meniscus that extends to the surface. AJR Am J Roentgenol 1993;161: 101–7.

[7] Tyrell RL, Gluckert K, Pathria M, et al. Fast three-dimensional MR imaging of the knee: a comparison with arthroscopy. Radiology 1988;166: 865–72.

[8] Ramnath RR. 3T MR imaging of the musculoskeletal system (Part 1): considerations, coils, and challenges. Magn Reson Imaging Clin N Am 2006;27–40.

[9] Gold GE, Han e, Stainsby J, et al. Musculoskeletal MRI at 3.0 T: relaxation times and image contrast. AJR Am J Roentgenol 2004;183:343–51.

[10] Gold GE, Suh B, Sawyer-Glover A, et al. Musculoskeletal MRI at 3.0 T: initial clinical experience. AJR Am J Roentgenol 2004;183:1479–86.

[11] Kaplan PA, Dussault R, Helms CA, et al. Knee. In: Kaplan PA, editor. Musculoskeletal MRI. Philadelphia: Saunders; 2001. p. 363–91.

[12] Magee T, Williams D. 3.0 T MRI of meniscal tears. AJR Am J Roentgenol 2006;187:371–5.

[13] Ramnath RR, Magee T, Wasudev N, et al. Accuracy of 3 T MRI using fast spin-echo technique to detect meniscal tears of the knee. AJR Am J Roentgenol 2006;187:221–5.

[14] Mosher TJ. Musculoskeletal imaging at 3T: current techniques and future applications. Magn Reson Imaging Clin N Am 2006;63–76.

RADIOLOGIC
CLINICS
OF NORTH AMERICA

Radiol Clin N Am 45 (2007) 1063–1068

Index

Note: Page numbers of article titles are in **boldface** type.

doi:10.1016/S0033-8389(07)00169-8

United States Postal Service
Statement of Ownership, Management, and Circulation
(All Periodicals Publications Except Requestor Publications)

1. Publication Title	2. Publication Number	3. Filing Date
Radiologic Clinics of North America	5 9 6 - 5 1 0	9/14/07

4. Issue Frequency	5. Number of Issues Published Annually	6. Annual Subscription Price
Jan, Mar, May, Jul, Sep, Nov	6	$259.00

7. Complete Mailing Address of Known Office of Publication (*Not printer*) (*Street, city, county, state, and ZIP+4*)

Elsevier Inc.
360 Park Avenue South
New York, NY 10010-1710

Contact Person: Stephen Bushing

Telephone (Include area code): 215-239-3688

8. Complete Mailing Address of Headquarters or General Business Office of Publisher (*Not printer*)

Elsevier Inc., 360 Park Avenue South, New York, NY 10010-1710

9. Full Names and Complete Mailing Addresses of Publisher, Editor, and Managing Editor (*Do not leave blank*)

Publisher (*Name and complete mailing address*)

John Schrefer, Elsevier, Inc., 1600 John F. Kennedy Blvd. Suite 1800, Philadelphia, PA 19103-2899

Editor (*Name and complete mailing address*)

Barton Dudlick, Elsevier, Inc., 1600 John F. Kennedy Blvd. Suite 1800, Philadelphia, PA 19103-2899

Managing Editor (*Name and complete mailing address*)

Catherine Bewick, Elsevier, Inc., 1600 John F. Kennedy Blvd. Suite 1800, Philadelphia, PA 19103-2899

10. Owner (*Do not leave blank. If the publication is owned by a corporation, give the name and address of the corporation immediately followed by the names and addresses of all stockholders owning or holding 1 percent or more of the total amount of stock. If not owned by a corporation, give the names and addresses of the individual owners. If owned by a partnership or other unincorporated firm, give its name and address as well as those of each individual owner. If the publication is published by a nonprofit organization, give its name and address.*)

Full Name	Complete Mailing Address
Wholly owned subsidiary of	4520 East-West Highway
Reed/Elsevier, US holdings	Bethesda, MD 20814

11. Known Bondholders, Mortgagees, and Other Security Holders Owning or Holding 1 Percent or More of Total Amount of Bonds, Mortgages, or Other Securities. If none, check box ☐ None

Full Name	Complete Mailing Address
N/A	

12. Tax Status (*For completion by nonprofit organizations authorized to mail at nonprofit rates*) (*Check one*)
The purpose, function, and nonprofit status of this organization and the exempt status for federal income tax purposes:
☐ Has Not Changed During Preceding 12 Months
☐ Has Changed During Preceding 12 Months (*Publisher must submit explanation of change with this statement*)

PS Form 3526, September 2006 (Page 1 of 3 (Instructions Page 3)) PSN 7530-01-000-9931 **PRIVACY NOTICE:** See our Privacy policy in www.usps.com

---

13. Publication Title	14. Issue Date for Circulation Data Below
Radiologic Clinics of North America	July 2007

15. Extent and Nature of Circulation		Average No. Copies Each Issue During Preceding 12 Months	No. Copies of Single Issue Published Nearest to Filing Date
a. Total Number of Copies (*Net press run*)		7550	7000
b. Paid Circulation (By Mail and Outside the Mail)	(1) Mailed Outside-County Paid Subscriptions Stated on PS Form 3541. (*Include paid distribution above nominal rate, advertiser's proof copies, and exchange copies*)	3834	3652
	(2) Mailed In-County Paid Subscriptions Stated on PS Form 3541 (*Include paid distribution above nominal rate, advertiser's proof copies, and exchange copies*)		
	(3) Paid Distribution Outside the Mails Including Sales Through Dealers and Carriers, Street Vendors, Counter Sales, and Other Paid Distribution Outside USPS®	2129	2131
	(4) Paid Distribution by Other Classes Mailed Through the USPS (e.g. First-Class Mail®)		
c. Total Paid Distribution (*Sum of 15b (1), (2), (3), and (4)*)	▲	5963	5783
d. Free or Nominal Rate Distribution (By Mail and Outside the Mail)	(1) Free or Nominal Rate Outside-County Copies Included on PS Form 3541	183	146
	(2) Free or Nominal Rate In-County Copies Included on PS Form 3541		
	(3) Free or Nominal Rate Copies Mailed at Other Classes Mailed Through the USPS (e.g. First-Class Mail)		
	(4) Free or Nominal Rate Distribution Outside the Mail (Carriers or other means)		
e. Total Free or Nominal Rate Distribution (Sum of 15d (1), (2), (3) and (4))		183	146
f. Total Distribution (Sum of 15c and 15e)	▲	6146	5929
g. Copies not Distributed (See instructions to publishers #4 (page #3))	▲	1404	1071
h. Total (Sum of 15f and g)	▲	7550	7000
i. Percent Paid (15c divided by 15f times 100)		97.02%	97.54%

16. Publication of Statement of Ownership
☐ If the publication is a general publication, publication of this statement is required. Will be printed in the November 2007 issue of this publication. ☐ Publication not required

17. Signature and Title of Editor, Publisher, Business Manager, or Owner

[signature] Adrian Fanucci – Executive Director of Subscription Services

Date: September 14, 2007

I certify that all information furnished on this form is true and complete. I understand that anyone who furnishes false or misleading information on this form or who omits material or information requested on the form may be subject to criminal sanctions (including fines and imprisonment) and/or civil sanctions (including civil penalties).

PS Form 3526, September 2006 (Page 2 of 3)

Moving?

Make sure your subscription moves with you!

To notify us of your new address, find your **Clinics Account Number** (located on your mailing label above your name), and contact customer service at:

E-mail: elspcs@elsevier.com

800-654-2452 (subscribers in the U.S. & Canada)
407-345-4000 (subscribers outside of the U.S. & Canada)

Fax number: 407-363-9661

Elsevier Periodicals Customer Service
6277 Sea Harbor Drive
Orlando, FL 32887-4800

*To ensure uninterrupted delivery of your subscription, please notify us at least 4 weeks in advance of move.